A Colour Handbook

Acute Adult Dermatology:
Diagnosis and Management

Daniel Creamer
Consultant Dermatologist, King's College Hospital, London, UK

Jonathan Barker
Professor of Clinical Dermatology, St. John's Institute of Dermatology,
King's College, London, UK

Francisco A Kerdel
Voluntary Professor and Director of Inpatient Dermatology,
University of Miami Hospital, Miami, Florida, USA

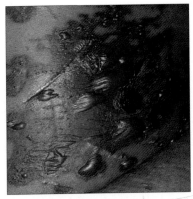

MANSON
PUBLISHING

Dedication

This book is dedicated to Katherine, Rebecca, and Patrick.

Copyright © 2011 Manson Publishing Ltd

ISBN: 978-1-84076-102-3

A CIP catalogue record for this book is available from the British Library.

For full details of all Manson Publishing titles please write to:
Manson Publishing Ltd, 73 Corringham Road, London NW11 7DL, UK.
Tel: +44(0)20 8905 5150
Fax: +44(0)20 8201 9233
Website: www.mansonpublishing.com

Commissioning editor: Jill Northcott
Project manager: Paul Bennett
Copy editor: Joanna Brocklesby
Layout: DiacriTech, Chennai, India
Colour reproduction: Tenon & Polert Colour Scanning Ltd, Hong Kong
Printed by: Finidr, s.r.o., Ceský Tesín, Czech Republic

Other Manson titles that may be of interest:
Chan: *Blistering Skin Diseases*
Elston: *Infectious Diseases of the Skin*
Ferguson & Dover: *Photodermatology*
Menter & Stoff: *Psoriasis*
Rycroft, Robertson & Wakelin: *Dermatology, A Colour Handbook*, 2nd edition
Sheridan: *Burns – A Practical Approach*

CONTENTS

Preface 5
Acknowledgements 6
Contributors 6

CHAPTER 1
Eczema 7
Atopic dermatitis 8
Eczema herpeticum 10
Pompholyx eczema 12
Discoid eczema 14
Venous eczema 16
Allergic and irritant contact
    dermatitis 18
Seborrhoeic dermatitis 20
Chronic actinic dermatitis . . . 22

CHAPTER 2
Psoriasis 25
Guttate psoriasis 26
Plaque psoriasis 28
Palmo-plantar pustulosis 30
Generalized pustular
    psoriasis 32

CHAPTER 3
Papular and papulo-
squamous dermatoses . . . 35
Lichen planus 36
Pityriasis rosea 38
Pityriasis rubra pilaris 40
Pityriasis lichenoides acuta . . 42
Eruptive xanthomata 44
Sarcoidosis 46
Darier's disease 48
Grover's disease 50

CHAPTER 4
Erythroderma 51

CHAPTER 5
Urticaria 55
Acute urticaria 56
Angio-oedema 58
The physical urticarias 60
Urticarial vasculitis 62

CHAPTER 6
Blistering diseases 65
Bullous pemphigoid 66
Pemphigus vulgaris and
    pemphigus foliaceous . . 68
Dermatitis herpetiformis . . . 72
Epidermolysis bullosa
    acquisita 74
Linear IgA bullous
    dermatosis 76
Porphyria cutanea tarda 78

CHAPTER 7
Vascular diseases 81
Small vessel vasculitis 82
Polyarteritis nodosa 84
Cutaneous embolism 86
Widespread cutaneous
    necrosis 88
Calciphylaxis 90
Pyoderma gangrenosum 92
Sweet's syndrome 94
Dependency syndrome 96

CHAPTER 8
Panniculitis 99
Erythema nodosum 100
Panniculitis 102

CHAPTER 9
Connective tissue
disease 105
Discoid lupus
    erythematosus 106
Systemic lupus
    erythematosus 108
Subacute cutaneous lupus
    erythematosus 110
Adult-onset Still's disease . . 112
Dermatomyositis 114

CHAPTER 10
Bacterial diseases 117
Impetigo 118
Folliculitis and
    furunculosis 120

Hidradenitis suppurativa . . . 122
Acne conglobata and acne
    fulminans 124
Erysipelas and cellulitis 126
Necrotizing fasciitis 128
Septic vasculitis
    and infectious purpura
    fulminans 130
Lyme disease 132
Toxic shock syndrome and
    staphylococcal scalded
    skin syndrome 134
Syphilis 136

CHAPTER 11
Viral diseases 139
Viral exanthem 140
Herpes simplex 142
Erythema multiforme 144
Chickenpox (varicella) 146
Herpes zoster (shingles) . . . 148
Orf 151

CHAPTER 12
Fungal diseases 153
Tinea (dermatophyte
    infections) 154
Candidiasis 158

CHAPTER 13
Dermatoses caused by
arthropods 161
Scabies 162
Insect bites 164
Pediculosis (lice) 166

CHAPTER 14
Travellers' and tropical
dermatoses 169
Cutaneous larva migrans . . 170
Furuncular myiasis 171
Tungiasis 172
Leishmaniasis 173
Onchocerciasis 174
Sporotrichosis 176
Rickettsial spotted fevers . . . 177

Dengue 178
Swimmer's itch 180
Sea-bathers' eruption 181
Jellyfish stings 182

CHAPTER 15
**Tumours and
malignancies** 185
Malignant melanoma 186
Squamous cell carcinoma . . 188
Pyogenic granuloma 191
Kaposi's sarcoma 192
Mycosis fungoides and
    Sézary syndrome 194
Primary cutaneous B cell
    lymphoma 196
Cutaneous metastases 198

CHAPTER 16
**Environmental and
physical dermatoses** 201
Chilblains 202
Miliaria 204
Minor burns 205
Dermatitis artefacta 206

Polymorphic light eruption . . 208
Phytophotodermatitis 210

CHAPTER 17
Pregnancy dermatoses . . 211
Polymorphic eruption of
    pregnancy 212
Pemphigoid gestationis 214

CHAPTER 18
**Drug- and therapy-induced
dermatoses** 217
Acute graft-versus-host
    disease 218
Drug-induced exanthem . . 220
Phototoxic drug eruption . . 222
Drug reaction with eosinophilia
    and systemic symptoms . . 224
Acute generalized
    exanthematous
    pustulosis 226
Fixed drug eruption 228
Stevens–Johnson
    syndrome/toxic
    epidermal necrolysis . . . 230

Abbreviations 235

Recommended reading . 236

Index 237

It is sometimes reckoned, by the ill-informed, that skin disease does not present acutely. This is quite untrue. A significant proportion of skin disease develops rapidly, is highly symptomatic, and can be associated with considerable morbidity. While most patients with acute skin disorders are initially seen by primary care services, 'hot' cases are also encountered in hospital emergency departments, and, of course, in dermatology clinics. However, for many of the clinicians who provide front-line medical care there is a relative lack of training in acute dermatology. This book aims to help meet that need.

In drawing up a list of conditions covered in this book two major criteria have been used: firstly, those dermatoses which are characterized by a sudden onset and rapid progression, and, secondly, diseases of the skin which are associated with significant local or systemic morbidity. The disorders presented include all the common inflammatory and infective dermatoses as well as a number of rarer conditions. There are also sections on tumours, connective tissue diseases, travellers' dermatoses, drug eruptions, and rashes caused by environmental and physical factors.

The presentation of a patient with an acute medical problem compels the clinician to supply an accurate diagnosis and an effective management plan quickly and efficiently. This demand is challenging in any branch of medicine. In the context of dermatology the clinician requires an ability to assess skin signs correctly coupled to a broad understanding of cutaneous disease and therapeutics. To optimize the consultation these virtues must be allied to a methodical clinical technique. Hopefully this book will provide a useful source of information as well as encouraging a structured and thorough approach to the patient with an acute dermatosis.

The sections have been written so that essential information about each disorder is summarized in a clear and concise way. After a brief introduction, there is a description of the clinical features, followed by a differential diagnosis, a list of important complications, and the relevant investigations. Treatment is divided into two sections, the first outlines the immediate action plan and the second highlights long-term management considerations. Each condition described is illustrated by clinical pictures.

It is hoped that this book will enable all medical staff seeing patients with acute skin problems to practise more effectively. It is aimed at dermatologists in training, primary care physicians, dermatology nurse specialists, and emergency department staff. It should also appeal to the general physician who is interested in dermatology.

Finally, as stated in the title, this is a book concerning adult skin disease. Although there is some overlap, acute dermatoses in neonates, infants, and children have a different clinical spectrum and often present in a contrasting way to adults. There is also a distinct approach to therapy in paediatric dermatology. These differences highlight the need for a separate book covering children's dermatoses and, at the time of writing, a companion volume entitled *Acute Paediatric Dermatology – A Colour Handbook* is in development.

Daniel Creamer
Jonathan Barker
Francisco A Kerdel

ACKNOWLEDGEMENTS

In writing this book I owe a great debt to my consultant colleagues, both past and present, in the department of dermatology at King's College Hospital, London; Dr Saqib Bashir, Dr Anthony du Vivier, Dr Claire Fuller, Prof Rod Hay, Dr Elisabeth Higgins, Dr Sarah Macfarlane, and Dr Rachael Morris-Jones. I have been lucky enough to benefit from their clinical experience and it is a pleasure to record my appreciation and thanks. It has also been my good fortune to collaborate with other colleagues on aspects of acute skin disease, and in particular I wish to acknowledge the help I obtained from Sister Judy Davids, Dr Patrick Gordon, Dr Nick Craven, and Mr Gregory Williams.

I would like to thank Prof Neil Cox who reviewed the manuscript and gave me some extremely helpful advice as I was flagging on the last lap.

The clinical images for this book have been supplied by the departments of medical photography at King's College Hospital and St John's Institute of Dermatology. I would like to thank the photographers from both departments for the superlative quality of their work. In particular I wish to thank Miss Lucy Wallace for her unflagging kindness in collating the images from King's. I also owe a special debt to Mr Stuart Robertson of the St John's Institute of Dermatology who has given his time and expertise so generously in the selection and preparation of all the pictures used. A few photographs have come from other sources and I wish to acknowledge the generosity of the following; Dr Lindsay Whittam, Dr Manuraj Singh, Dr Andrew Pembroke, Mr Gregory Williams, Dr Sheena Allan, Dr Ruth MacSween.

An educational grant from Leo Pharma helped towards preparing the book images and I am extremely grateful to them for supporting this project.

Finally it is a pleasure to acknowledge the unfailing help and extreme patience of Ms Jill Northcott of Manson Publishing.

CONTRIBUTORS

The following doctors contributed sections to the book while they were undertaking their training in dermatology:

Karim Amin, Saqib Bashir, Emma Benton, Samantha Bunting, Ai-Lean Chew, Emma Craythorne, Simon Dawe, Paul Farrant, Sacha Goolamali, Justine Hextall, Sharon Jacobs, Sarah Macfarlane, Claire Martyn-Simmons, Lesley-Ann Murphy, Jana Natkunarajah, Nuala O'Donoghue, Guy Perera, Laura Proudfoot, Sandrine Reynaert, James Shelley, Kate Short, Karen Watson, Jonathan White, Juliet Williams, Sharon Wong, Tracey Wong.

Eczema

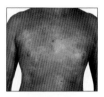 Atopic dermatitis

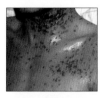 Eczema herpeticum

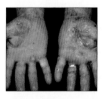 Pompholyx eczema

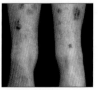 Discoid eczema

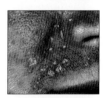 Venous eczema

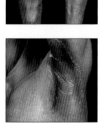 Allergic and irritant contact dermatitis

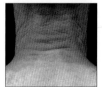 Seborrhoeic dermatitis

 Chronic actinic dermatitis

Atopic dermatitis

In atopic dermatitis (AD) the skin is chronically dry and itchy but also susceptible to intermittent inflammatory exacerbations. An acute flare of AD is characterized by worsening pruritus and active skin inflammation which, if untreated, can involve the whole skin. A number of factors can precipitate an exacerbation of AD, including temperature changes (central heating), strong sunlight (in some individuals, in others summer sunshine is helpful), common allergens (house dust mite, animal dander), and pregnancy. Secondary staphylococcal skin infection commonly complicates acute AD and, indeed, may be the trigger for a sudden deterioration in previously well controlled eczema.

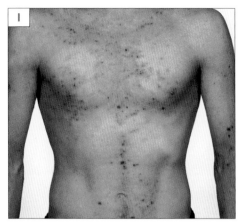

1 Atopic dermatitis. This patient's skin was intensely itchy. There are numerous excoriated papules on a background of patchy erythema.

CLINICAL FEATURES

Examination of active AD reveals areas of poorly defined erythema, inflammatory papules, and fine scaling (**1**). The sites of predilection are the face, neck, limb flexures, and hands (**2**). When very active the erythema of AD is urticated and can rapidly spread to involve the whole skin (**3**). The intense itch leads to scratching which results in linear scratch marks and excoriated papules (**4**). White dermographism describes pale streaks from scratching within areas of erythema. Unlike other forms of acute dermatitis, vesicles do not occur in active AD, however a serous exudate and crusting may be present. Secondary bacterial infection with *Staphylococcus aureus* causes a honey-coloured discolouration to the scale (impetiginization) (**5**). Patients with long-standing AD also display the signs of chronic eczema, such as lichenification.

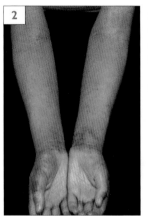

2 Atopic dermatitis. Fixed erythema is a sign of active AD. Flexural surfaces are commonly involved.

DIFFERENTIAL DIAGNOSIS
- Seborrhoeic dermatitis (p. 20, erythema and scaling of the face, scalp, and chest).
- Contact dermatitis (p. 18, eczema in a localized area or unusual distribution).
- Eczema herpeticum (p. 10, eczema plus small, punched-out erosions of herpes simplex virus (HSV) infection).
- Scabies infestation (p. 162, severe pruritus plus burrows at the wrists and finger webs).

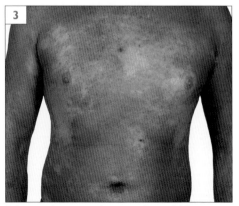

3 Atopic dermatitis. An acute flare of AD can result in extensive areas of urticated erythema.

COMPLICATIONS
- Malaise and fatigue (with extensive involvement).
- Regional lymphadenopathy (with secondary bacterial infection).
- Fever (with severe secondary bacterial infection).
- Erythroderma (see p. 51).

INVESTIGATIONS
- The diagnosis is usually made clinically.
- Skin swab for bacteriology (*S. aureus* infection occurs commonly).
- Skin swab for virology (if secondary infection with HSV is suspected).
- Swab of anterior nares for bacteriology (to exclude nasal carriage of *S. aureus*).
- Blood count, basic chemistry, liver function tests (if considering systemic immunosuppressant therapy or if the patient is systemically unwell).

IMMEDIATE MANAGEMENT
Topical therapy
- General emollient therapy.
- Corticosteroid ointment, twice per day (use for a restricted period):
    face: mildly potent.
    trunk and limbs: moderately potent.
- A gauze bodysuit can be used to maximize the effects of topical therapy.

Systemic therapy
- For secondary bacterial infection give antistaphylococcal oral antibiotics (e.g. flucloxacillin 500 mg four times per day for 7 days).
- A sedating oral antihistamine at bedtime (e.g. hydroxyzine 25 or 50 mg) will relieve itch and improve sleep.
- A short, reducing course of oral corticosteroids can be helpful to induce remission (e.g. prednisolone 20–30 mg/day and reducing by 5 mg every 5th day).

LONG-TERM MANAGEMENT ISSUES
Adherence to appropriate skin care is essential to maintain a remission: regular use of an emollient, bath oil, and soap substitute is essential. Other conservative measures should be considered: cotton clothing, the control of house dust mite in the home, and behaviour modification techniques to prevent scratching. Nasal carriage of *S. aureus* needs to be treated with fusidic acid or mupiricin ointment or chlorhexidine cream applied to the anterior nares three times per day for 7 days. Intermittent use of topical corticosteroid or immunomodulator (e.g. tacrolimus, pimecrolimus) is usually necessary. Patients with severe, recalcitrant AD need to be under the care of a dermatologist and may require treatment with second-line therapy, such as phototherapy or systemic immunosuppressants (e.g. azathioprine or ciclosporin).

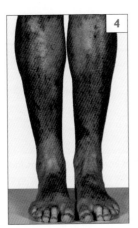

4 Atopic dermatitis. Repeated scratching aggravates inflammation, produces excoriations, and increases the likelihood of secondary infection.

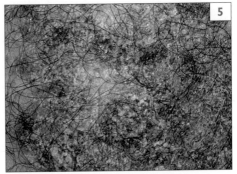

5 Impetiginized atopic dermatitis. Golden or honey-coloured crusts overlying eczema indicate secondary infection with *S. aureus*.

Eczema herpeticum

Eczema herpeticum is the widespread infection of atopic dermatitis by herpes simplex virus (HSV). It can occur in an atopic dermatitis patient who develops a cold sore or who comes into contact with an active herpetic lesion on another individual. This condition, with the alternative name of Kaposi's varicelliform eruption, can also occur in cutaneous T cell lymphoma, pemphigus foliaceous, and Darier's disease. Less commonly it can occur following genital HSV infection. Eczema herpeticum is a serious dermatosis which can progress into a disseminated and potentially fatal systemic herpetic infection.

CLINICAL FEATURES

Secondary herpetic infection of eczema can be difficult to identify and should therefore be considered in all patients with an acute flare of atopic dermatitis. The eruption of eczema herpeticum is painful and usually involves the face, neck, and upper chest, but can become widely disseminated. It is characterized by discrete vesicles and vesico-pustules occurring on red, eczematous skin which burst to leave punctate, haemorrhagic erosions (**6**). Coalescence of individual lesions produces large eroded areas (**7**). During the acute phase there may be significant local oedema. Lesional skin may become additionally infected with *S. aureus* or streptococci. The associated impetiginized crust may obscure the signs of herpes infection (**8**).

DIFFERENTIAL DIAGNOSIS
- Impetiginized atopic dermatitis (p. 8, eczema with overlying honey-coloured crust).
- Impetigo (p. 118, areas of erythema with superficial blisters and overlying honey-coloured crust).
- Primary HSV infection (p. 142, cluster of vesicles on a red base).
- Primary varicella zoster virus (VZV) infection (chicken pox) (p. 146, disseminated vesicles, each on a red macule).

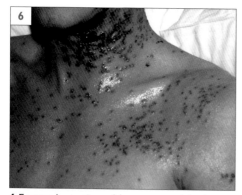

6 Eczema herpeticum. Numerous vesicles have ruptured to produce circular erosions. Eczema herpeticum usually occurs on the face or neck.

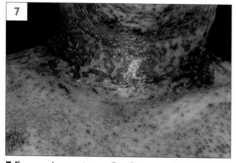

7 Eczema herpeticum. Confluence of numerous individual herpetic lesions can result in a large eroded area often with straight or angulated margins.

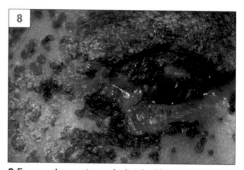

8 Eczema herpeticum. Individual lesions on the temple and lower eyelid can be seen but extensive impetiginized crust on the upper eyelid and eyebrow has obscured signs of herpetic infection.

COMPLICATIONS
- Fever (if infection is severe).
- Malaise.
- Regional lymphadenopathy.
- Hepatitis.
- Pneumonitis.
- Encephalitis.

INVESTIGATIONS
- Skin swab of vesicle base for viral culture (culture of HSV from vesicle fluid takes 1–5 days).
- Collection of vesicle fluid and scrapings of ulcer base for immunofluorescence, electron microscopy, and polymerase chain reaction (PCR) (electron microscopy can identify viruses of the herpes family rapidly; immunofluorescence of vesicle scrapings can differentiate HSV1 and HSV2; HSV PCR is the most sensitive identification method).
- Tzanck smear: scrapings of the ulcer base for cytology (a nonspecific test demonstrating multinucleated giant cells and intranuclear inclusion bodies in epithelial cells).
- Skin swab for bacteriology (if secondary bacterial infection is suspected).
- Blood count, basic chemistry, liver function tests (if patient is systemically unwell).
- Chest radiograph (to exclude herpes pneumonitis).

IMMEDIATE MANAGEMENT
Topical therapy
- General emollient therapy.
- Potassium permanganate soaks once per day.

Systemic therapy
- For modest involvement, with no systemic features: oral aciclovir 200 mg five times per day for 5 days. An alternative to aciclovir is valaciclovir 500 mg twice per day for 5 days.
- For moderate or severe involvement, or any case with systemic features: intravenous aciclovir 5 mg/kg three times per day for 5 days (10 mg/kg three times per day for 5 days in the immuno-compromised).

- With concomitant staphylococcal or streptococcal infection give oral or intravenous antibiotics.

Supportive therapy
Patients with moderate or severe eczema herpeticum should be admitted to hospital for the following:
- Bed rest and intensive topical therapy (see above).
- Monitoring of vital signs (pulse rate, blood pressure, temperature).
- Monitoring of fluid balance and administration of intravenous fluids, if required.
- Initiation of systemic therapy (see above).
- Analgesia.

LONG-TERM MANAGEMENT ISSUES
Following treatment, the erosions of eczema herpeticum generally heal within 1–2 weeks. Once the herpetic infection has been treated, manage the underlying atopic dermatitis with topical therapy (see Atopic dermatitis, p. 8). Ensuring the dermatitis is well controlled is essential in minimizing any future risk of reinfection with HSV. Patients with atopic dermatitis should have cold sores treated aggressively and should avoid close contact with an individual who has an open cold sore. In recurrent HSV infections consider giving prophylactic oral aciclovir 400 mg twice per day for 6 months.

Pompholyx eczema

Pompholyx or dyshidrotic eczema is characterized by vesicles on the palms and soles. The hands are more commonly affected than the feet but both sites may be involved concurrently. Although pompholyx eczema appears to be a distinct entity it may represent a manifestation of atopy or a presentation of contact dermatitis. Palmar pompholyx also occurs as a response to dermatophyte infection of the feet (tinea pedis). The vesiculation and blistering of pompholyx eczema often develops suddenly and, because of the sites of involvement, can be functionally disabling.

CLINICAL FEATURES

Deep-seated, itchy vesicles develop on the palms and lateral borders of the fingers and on the soles of the feet (**9, 10**). The signs are usually symmetrical. Unlike other forms of eczema there is little associated dryness in the acute phase. Coalescence of individual vesicles can produce large tense blisters, especially on the feet. Rupture of the blisters will lead to weeping and sometimes secondary staphylococcal or streptococcal infection. Attacks usually subside spontaneously after a few weeks with desquamation.

DIFFERENTIAL DIAGNOSIS

- Contact dermatitis (p. 18, eczema in localized area or unusual distribution).
- Palmo-plantar pustulosis (p. 30, pustules on palms and soles with scaling).
- Bullous tinea manum/pedis (p. 154, unilateral itchy blisters with erythema on palms or soles).

COMPLICATIONS

- Regional lymphadenopathy (with secondary bacterial infection).
- Erysipelas/cellulitis.

INVESTIGATIONS

- The diagnosis is usually made clinically.
- Swabs for bacteriology (if secondary infection is suspected).
- Skin scrapings for mycology (to exclude dermatophyte infection).
- Patch testing (if allergic contact dermatitis is suspected).

IMMEDIATE MANAGEMENT
Topical therapy
- General emollient therapy.
- Potassium permanganate soaks once per day after rupturing blisters.
- Corticosteroid ointment, twice per day (use for a restricted period):
  palms and soles: potent.
  (Corticosteroid efficacy can be enhanced by occlusion using polythene gloves for the hands and plastic kitchen wrap for the feet.)

Systemic therapy
- For secondary bacterial infection give antistaphylococcal oral antibiotics (e.g. flucloxacillin 500 mg four times per day for 7 days).
- In severe involvement a short course of oral corticosteroids can be helpful to induce a remission (e.g. prednisolone 20–30 mg/day and reducing by 5 mg every 5th day).

LONG-TERM MANAGEMENT ISSUES

Adherence to appropriate skin care is essential to maintain a remission: regular use of an emollient and soap substitute is essential. Hyperhidrosis can be a contributory factor in plantar pompholyx eczema, therefore careful foot hygiene and iontophoresis may be helpful. Patch testing must be performed in patients with chronic pompholyx eczema to exclude an allergic contact dermatitis. Severe, recalcitrant pompholyx eczema may respond to hand–foot phototherapy, systemic retinoid (e.g. acitretin), or systemic immunosuppressants (e.g. azathioprine or ciclosporin).

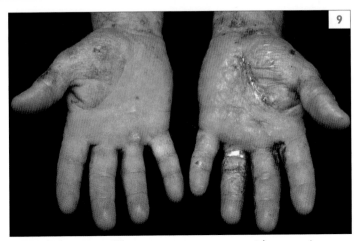

9 Pompholyx eczema. There are numerous tense vesicles occurring on the skin of the palms, worst on the left. In places the vesicles have become confluent.

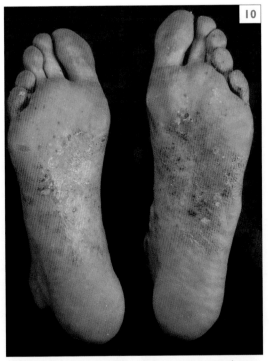

10 Pompholyx eczema. There is extensive vesiculation on the soles of the feet. Some lesions have become pustular indicating secondary infection with *S. aureus*.

Discoid eczema

Discoid (or nummular) eczema is characterized by discrete, round patches of dermatitis. Sometimes a solitary lesion will occur, more commonly they are multiple. The eruption is very itchy and often develops suddenly, precipitating an acute presentation.

CLINICAL FEATURES

In discoid eczema a localized area of dermatitis initially develops on the lower aspect of one leg (**11**). The lesion starts as a cluster of tiny papules which become confluent and evolve into an intensely itchy, disc-shaped patch or plaque (**12**). Thereafter several similar, discoid lesions may appear elsewhere on the legs and arms. In severe cases, patches of eczema can also develop on the torso (**13**). Initially the lesions are weepy but become dry with time, often covered by an impetiginized crust.

DIFFERENTIAL DIAGNOSIS

- Tinea corporis (p. 154, annular lesions with inflammatory margins).
- Plaque psoriasis (p. 28, scaly plaques distributed symmetrically, typical nail changes).
- Bowen's disease (intraepidermal carcinoma: red patch with mild scale and distinct margin).
- Mycosis fungoides (p. 194, pink or red patches with superficial atrophy, distributed asymmetrically).

COMPLICATIONS

There are usually none.

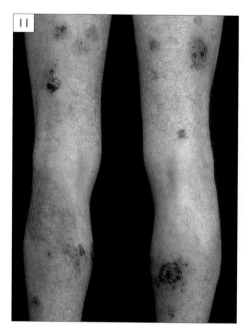

11 Discoid eczema. Involvement of the legs is typical, often multiple lesions develop.

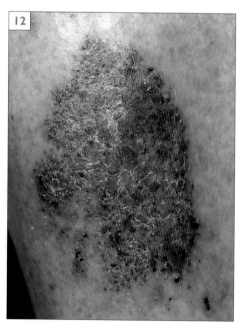

12 Discoid eczema. Individual lesions are oval or circular and well circumscribed.

INVESTIGATIONS
- The diagnosis is usually made clinically.
- Skin swab for bacteriology (if secondary infection is suspected).
- Skin scrapings for mycology (to exclude dermatophyte infection).
- Skin biopsy for histopathology if the diagnosis is in doubt (epidermal spongiosis, vesiculation, acanthosis, and exocytosis of lymphocytes and neutrophils).

IMMEDIATE MANAGEMENT
Topical therapy
- General emollient therapy.
- Corticosteroid ointment, twice per day (use for a restricted period):
    trunk and limbs: potent.
    (Corticosteroid efficacy can be enhanced by occlusion using a dressing or a tubular bandage.)

Systemic therapy
- For extensive secondary bacterial infection give antistaphylococcal oral antibiotics (e.g. flucloxacillin 500 mg four times per day for 7 days).

LONG-TERM MANAGEMENT ISSUES
Discoid eczema tends to run a chronic course and consequently prolonged adherence to appropriate skin care is essential. Relapses can be treated with topical therapy, as above. Severe recalcitrant discoid eczema may respond to phototherapy or systemic immunosuppressants (e.g. azathioprine, ciclosporin). In some cases chronic discoid eczema may be associated with alcohol misuse and, therefore, advice on alcohol restriction can be helpful. Patients with chronic discoid eczema or who suffer frequent relapses should undergo patch tests to exclude an allergic contact dermatitis.

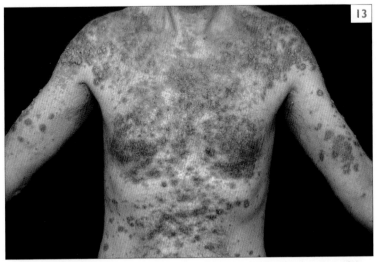

13 Discoid eczema. In severe discoid eczema there may be involvement of the arms and torso, as with this patient. In areas there is an extensive impetiginized crust, indicating heavy secondary infection with S. aureus.

Venous eczema

Venous eczema involves the skin of the lower legs and develops as a result of venous insufficiency. It tends to occur in elderly patients with venous incompetence arising from varicose veins or previous deep venous thrombosis (DVT). The eruption may develop acutely and, if unilateral, can be mistaken for cellulitis.

CLINICAL FEATURES

Initially there is erythema involving the medial aspect of the lower leg (**14**). The eruption is very itchy and usually becomes excoriated (**15**). With time venous eczema extends to involve the whole of the lower leg and foot. Scaling and crusting is often prominent. There are usually other signs of venous insufficiency, e.g. varicose veins, oedema, haemosiderin deposition, lipodermatosclerosis, and ulceration. Autosens-itization can occur in which papular eczema appears on the arms and torso as a reactive phenomenon to eczema on the legs. As with other forms of dermatitis, venous eczema can be complicated by secondary bacterial infection.

DIFFERENTIAL DIAGNOSIS

- Allergic contact dermatitis (p. 18, eczema in a localized area or unusual distribution).
- Dependency syndrome (p. 96, lymphoedema and venous congestion in poorly mobile, chair-bound individuals).
- Discoid eczema (p. 14, discrete, oval patches of eczema, usually on lower legs).
- Psoriasis (p. 28, scaly plaques distributed symmetrically, typical nail changes).
- Erysipelas/cellulitis (p. 126, zone of painful, spreading erythema with fever).

COMPLICATIONS
- Erysipelas/cellulitis.

INVESTIGATIONS
- The diagnosis is usually made clinically.
- Skin swabs for bacteriology (if secondary infection is suspected).
- Venous studies (may identify a cause for venous insufficiency, e.g. perforator incompetence, past DVT).
- Ankle–brachial pressure index (ABPI) of affected leg (ABPI <0.8 indicates significant arterial disease and compression should be avoided).
- Thrombophilia screen with history of DVT (to exclude clotting diathesis).

IMMEDIATE MANAGEMENT
Topical therapy
- General emollient therapy.
- Corticosteroid ointment, twice per day (use for a restricted period):
    legs: potent.
- Leg elevation.

Systemic therapy
- For secondary bacterial infection give antistaphylococcal oral antibiotics (e.g. flucloxacillin 500 mg four times per day for 7 days).

LONG-TERM MANAGEMENT ISSUES
Venous eczema tends to run a chronic course and therefore adherence to appropriate skin care is essential. Compression bandaging can be helpful to induce remission. Long-term use of support hosiery can prevent relapses. A vascular surgical opinion may be helpful to identify any correctible venous disorder. If the eczema fails to remit with appropriate treatment then consider a secondary allergic contact dermatitis to medicaments in topical agents or to rubber in elasticated bandages or hosiery.

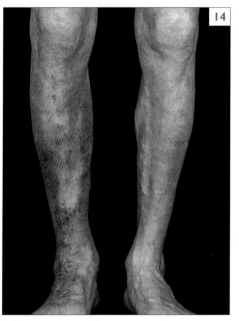

14 Venous eczema. This patient with varicose veins, worse on the right, has venous eczema involving the right lower leg.

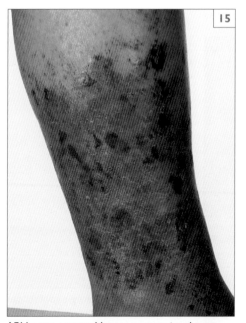

15 Venous eczema. Venous eczema involves the gaiter area of the lower leg. It often gets excoriated.

Allergic and irritant contact dermatitis

Contact dermatitis is an eczema caused by skin contact with an exogenous substance. It is divided into two groups: (1) allergic contact dermatitis (ACD), which is a delayed hypersensitivity reaction to an exogenous allergen; (2) irritant contact dermatitis (ICD), which is induced by direct inflammatory pathways without prior sensitization. Certain occupations are considered more likely to predispose individuals to develop contact dermatitis, e.g. hairdressing, cleaning, catering, nursing, child care, and construction. Common sensitizers include nickel in jewellery, rubber in gloves and shoes, and preservatives in cosmetics. Identification of the relevant allergen requires information concerning the relation of the dermatitis with work, periods away from work (e.g. holidays), hobbies, and household chores. Severe ACD can occur in patients allergic to certain plants, e.g. poison ivy. Some substances are photoallergens and need both sunlight and the chemical to induce dermatitis. In ICD the common irritants include detergents, water, organic solvents, acidic and alkaline chemicals. Contact dermatitis can present acutely, often in an individual with no previous history of eczema.

CLINICAL FEATURES

Acute contact dermatitis of both types is characterized by erythema, oedema, vesicles, and exudation. The precise distribution of the eruption may provide a valuable diagnostic clue to the likely allergen or irritant (**16–19**). For example, involvement of ear lobes may suggest ACD to nickel in jewellery, involvement of the face may suggest ACD to preservatives or fragrances in skin-care products. With prolonged exposure to an allergen the dermatitis will extend beyond the zone of contact. In ICD the hands are the sites most usually affected, both dorsal and palmar surfaces, often secondary to prolonged contact with irritants such as detergent and water. Mild irritants cause redness, dryness, and scaling, whereas potent irritants induce fiery erythema, oedema, vesicles, and, in some cases, ulceration.

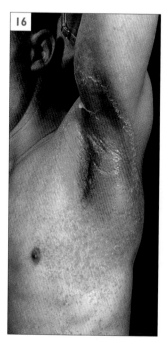

16 Allergic contact dermatitis. There is an extensive zone of acute eczema in the axilla. This patient was allergic to a preservative in his deodorant.

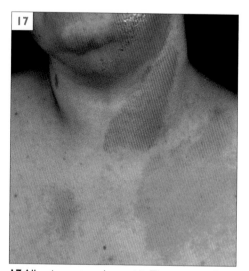

17 Allergic contact dermatitis. There are well demarcated patches of erythema and swelling on the cheek, neck, and chest. The patient was allergic to a component of her boyfriend's topical acne treatment.

DIFFERENTIAL DIAGNOSIS

Face
- Atopic dermatitis (p. 8, eczema as part of atopic diathesis).
- Seborrhoeic dermatitis (p. 20, erythema and scaling of the face, scalp, and chest).
- Psoriasis (p. 25, scaly plaques distributed symmetrically, typical nail changes).
- Tinea facei (p. 154, annular lesion(s) with inflammatory margin).

Hands
- Atopic dermatitis (p. 8, eczema as part of atopic diathesis).
- Psoriasis (p. 28, scaly plaques distributed symmetrically, typical nail changes).
- Pompholyx eczema (p. 12, vesicular eczema of palmo-plantar skin).
- Tinea manum (p. 154, erythema and scaling, usually affecting one hand only).

Feet and lower legs
- Venous eczema (p. 16, eczema on lower legs caused by venous insufficiency).
- Psoriasis (p. 28, scaly plaques distributed symmetrically, typical nail changes).
- Pompholyx eczema (p. 12, vesicular eczema of palmo-plantar skin).
- Tinea pedis (p. 154, erythema and scaling of foot (feet), usually involving toe web(s)).

COMPLICATIONS
- Regional lymphadenopathy (with secondary bacterial infection).
- Erysipelas/cellulitis (rare).

INVESTIGATIONS
- Patch tests (multiple, standardized allergens are applied to the upper back: a positive reaction confirms an allergic contact sensitivity; multiple allergens in a single patient is common).
- Skin swabs for bacteriology (if secondary infection is suspected).

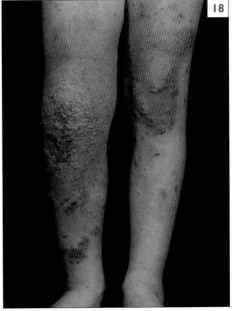

18 Allergic contact dermatitis. This patient has acute dermatitis, worse on the right leg, with erythema, vesiculation, swelling, and impetiginization. This was triggered by contact with poison ivy.

19 Allergic contact dermatitis. ACD to a topical analgesic applied to the lower leg under a bandage. There has been a blistering reaction with an area of epidermal loss over the calf. The sharp cut-off denotes the zone of analgesic application and the limits of the bandage.

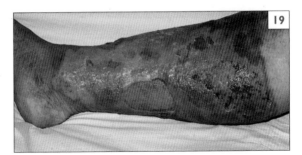

IMMEDIATE MANAGEMENT
Topical therapy
- ICD: following recent contact with a potent chemical irritant, lavage immediately with water.
- ACD: identify potential allergen and avoid further contact.
- General emollient therapy.
- Corticosteroid ointment, twice per day (use for a restricted period):
  face: moderately potent.
  trunk and limbs: potent.
- If vesiculation and weeping are prominent use potassium permanganate soaks once per day.

Systemic therapy
- For secondary bacterial infection give antistaphylococcal oral antibiotics (e.g. flucloxacillin 500 mg four times per day for 7 days).
- With severe contact dermatitis give a short course of oral corticosteroids (e.g. prednisolone 20–30 mg/day and reducing by 5 mg every 5th day).

LONG-TERM MANAGEMENT ISSUES
Careful interpretation of patch tests by a dermatologist is central to the correct management of a patient with ACD. Once initial sensitization to an allergen has occurred the potential to react persists indefinitely and continued exposure to the allergen will result in chronic ACD. It is therefore important that information concerning sources of allergen exposure is given to the patient. Long-term skin care with the regular use of an emollient is helpful in prolonging remission. The use of topical tacrolimus ointment or pimecrolimus cream will reduce requirements for topical corticosteroid. In ICD persistence of contact with irritant will induce dryness, scaling, and lichenification. Avoidance of the irritant(s) will eventually facilitate resolution of the dermatitis. In ICD the use of relevant protective clothing and barrier creams can be helpful. Patients with irritant hand dermatitis must be encouraged to wear vinyl gloves when undertaking wet work.

Seborrhoeic dermatitis

Seborrhoeic dermatitis occurs at sites rich in sebaceous glands and is caused by an excess of *Malassezia* yeasts in these areas. Seborrhoeic dermatitis tends to run a relapsing–remitting course, however acute exacerbations are common.

CLINICAL FEATURES
The scalp is almost always involved with itchy erythema and scaling causing dandruff. On the face, areas of predilection include the hairline, eyebrows, glabella, and nasolabial folds (**20, 21**). Blepharitis is common. Involvement of the presternal and flexural skin is characterized by well demarcated patches of erythema with scaling. An acute, severe flare can result in widespread eczema with minimal scaling involving the head, face, neck, torso, and flexures (**22**).

DIFFERENTIAL DIAGNOSIS
- Psoriasis (p. 27, scaly plaques distributed symmetrically, typical nail changes).
- Contact dermatitis (p. 18, eczema in a localized area or unusual distribution).
- Atopic dermatitis (p. 8, eczema as part of the atopic diathesis).
- Tinea faciale/corporis (p. 154, annular lesions with inflammatory margins).
- Subacute cutaneous lupus erythematosus (p. 110, annular and polycyclic rash on torso).

COMPLICATIONS
There are usually none.

INVESTIGATIONS
- The diagnosis is usually made clinically.

IMMEDIATE MANAGEMENT
Topical therapy
- General emollient therapy.
- Treat scalp involvement with ketoconazole shampoo.
- Corticosteroid ointment, twice per day (use for a restricted period):
    - face and flexures: mildly potent containing azole antifungal.
    - torso and limbs: moderately potent.

LONG-TERM MANAGEMENT ISSUES
Seborrhoeic dermatitis tends to relapse and so active therapy may need to be reinstated intermittently. Long-term skin care with the regular use of an emollient is helpful in prolonging remission. The use of topical tacrolimus ointment or pimecrolimus cream will reduce requirements for topical corticosteroid. For unresponsive cases a course of oral itraconazole (200 mg once daily for 14 days) can be useful. Ultraviolet B (UVB) phototherapy may also be helpful. In some cases seborrhoeic dermatitis can be associated with alcohol misuse and, therefore, advice on alcohol restriction may be useful. HIV infection should be considered in patients with extensive and poorly controlled seborrhoeic dermatitis.

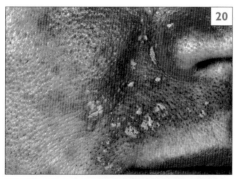

20 Seborrhoeic dermatitis. Involvement of the nasolabial folds with erythema and scaling is typical.

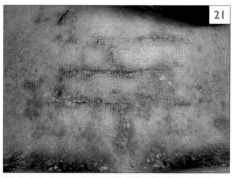

21 Seborrhoeic dermatitis. The forehead and eyebrows are common sites of involvement.

22 Seborrhoeic dermatitis. In severe, acute seborrhoeic dermatitis widespread involvement can occur on the torso. This patient was found to have HIV infection.

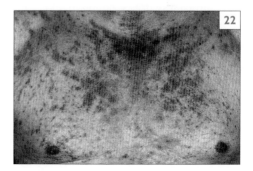

Chronic actinic dermatitis

Chronic actinic dermatitis (CAD) is a rare form of eczema induced by sunlight and is seen most commonly in middle-aged or elderly men. Although affected individuals have abnormal photosensitivity the causative role of sunlight is sometimes not immediately apparent to the patient. The dermatitis develops on exposed skin, occurring maximally during the spring and summer months when the ultraviolet component of sunshine is high. Most patients are sensitive to UVB radiation but also to ultraviolet A (UVA) and, in some cases, visible light. Despite its name, CAD can present acutely as a clinically striking and highly symptomatic dermatosis.

CLINICAL FEATURES

CAD is characterized by eczema involving the light-exposed sites: face, neck, upper chest, and back of hands (**23, 24, 25**). Usually the limits of clothing (collar and cuffs) produce a clear cut-off with the covered skin being unaffected (**24, 25**). Involved skin shows confluent eczema although there will be sparing in light-protected areas such as finger webs, upper eyelids, and the submental zone. Although the signs may suggest a chronic form of eczema (lichenification, induration, and scaling), CAD can present as a subacute or acute dermatitis with erythema, swelling, weeping, and secondary infection. In severe cases the eczema may spread from exposed skin to covered sites and lead to erythroderma.

DIFFERENTIAL DIAGNOSIS

- Allergic contact dermatitis (p. 18, eczema in a localized area or unusual distribution).
- Airborne allergic contact dermatitis (p. 18, eczema localized to the exposed skin).
- Photosensitive drug eruption (p. 222, erythema on exposed skin triggered by a photosensitizing drug).
- Photoaggravated atopic dermatitis (p. 8, atopic dermatitis exacerbated by sunlight).
- Photoaggravated seborrhoeic dermatitis (p. 20, seborrhoeic dermatitis exacerbated by sunlight).

COMPLICATIONS

- Regional lymphadenopathy (with secondary bacterial infection).
- Erythroderma (see p. 51).

INVESTIGATIONS

- The diagnosis is usually made clinically.
- Skin swab for bacteriology (if secondary bacterial infection is suspected).
- Blood count, basic chemistry, liver function tests (needed if considering systemic immunosuppressant therapy or if the patient is systemically unwell).
- Antinuclear antibody (ANA), -Ro and -La antibodies (to exclude lupus-related photosensitivity).
- Diagnostic light tests: monochromator irradiation testing and solar simulator testing (these tests, performed in a specialist photobiology unit, will confirm the diagnosis and identify the provoking wavelengths of light).
- Patch tests (many patients with CAD also have positive patch tests, especially to plant allergens, suggesting concomitant allergic contact dermatitis).

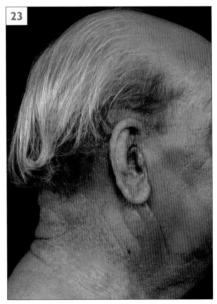

23 Chronic actinic dermatitis. There is eczema involving all the exposed skin of the face and scalp with a cut-off at the neck, caused by the patient's collar.

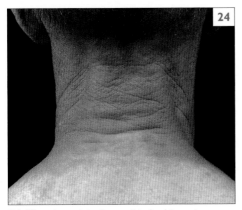

24 Chronic actinic dermatitis. In this patient with CAD there is a distinct demarcation between the covered, unaffected skin of the back and the exposed, eczematous skin of the neck.

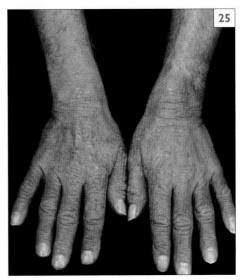

25 Chronic actinic dermatitis. There are florid eczematous changes on the backs of the hands, less severe involvement on the forearms, and sparing under the watch.

IMMEDIATE MANAGEMENT
Topical therapy
- Sun avoidance and use of photoprotective clothing, including a broad-brimmed hat.
- Use of high protection factor topical sunscreen containing effective UVA and UVB filters.
- General emollient therapy.
- Corticosteroid ointment, twice per day (use for a restricted period):
    face: moderately potent.
    neck, arms, hands: potent.

Systemic therapy
- For secondary bacterial infection give antistaphylococcal oral antibiotics (e.g. flucloxacillin 500 mg four times per day for 7 days).
- A sedating oral antihistamine at bedtime (e.g. hydroxyzine 25 or 50 mg) will relieve itch and improve sleep.
- A short, reducing course of oral corticosteroids can be helpful to induce a remission (e.g. prednisolone 20–30 mg/day and reducing by 5 mg every 5th day).

LONG-TERM MANAGEMENT ISSUES
Ongoing attention to photoprotection is essential and CAD patients usually need long-term follow-up by a dermatologist. Patients who are sensitive to the longer wavelengths of UVA and visible light may require special filters on the glass of windows at home and in their car. CAD tends to relapse each spring and summer and therefore active therapy may need to be reinstated seasonally. Topical tacrolimus ointment or pimecrolimus cream may reduce requirements for topical or oral corticosteroid. Patients with severe CAD or those who are extremely photosensitive will require long-term systemic immunosuppression with azathioprine or ciclosporin. If patch tests are positive patients should be encouraged to avoid relevant allergens. There is a rare association between CAD and HIV infection.

Psoriasis

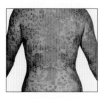 **Guttate psoriasis**

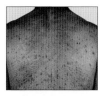 **Plaque psoriasis**

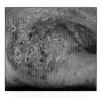 **Palmo-plantar pustulosis**

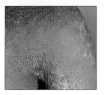 **Generalized pustular psoriasis**

Guttate psoriasis

Guttate psoriasis is an eruptive form of psoriasis which tends to affect young adults and often follows an episode of streptococcal pharyngitis. Typically the eruption is widespread and develops suddenly causing the patient to seek an urgent opinion.

CLINICAL FEATURES

There are numerous red papules and small plaques measuring 2–10 mm in diameter disseminated over the body, particularly on the trunk and proximal limbs (**26, 27**). Initially scaling is minimal but as the lesions increase in size surface hyperkeratosis develops. Guttate psoriasis can be itchy but is often asymptomatic. The patient may give a history of a sore throat 10–14 days prior to the appearance of skin lesions.

DIFFERENTIAL DIAGNOSIS

- Pityriasis rosea (p. 38, an eruption of slightly scaly patches following an initial 'herald' lesion).
- Secondary syphilis (p. 136, a papulo-squamous eruption with acral involvement).
- Lichen planus (p. 36, violaceous papules and plaques, typical changes in the mouth).

COMPLICATIONS

There are usually none.

INVESTIGATIONS

- The diagnosis is usually made clinically.
- Throat swab (to identify streptococcal infection).
- Streptococcal serology (as above).

IMMEDIATE MANAGEMENT
Topical therapy

- General emollient therapy.
- Corticosteroid ointment, twice per day (use for a restricted period):
  trunk and limbs: moderately potent.
- UVB phototherapy.

Systemic therapy

- Treat pharyngitis with oral antibiotics (e.g. penicillin V 500 mg four times per day for 7 days).

LONG-TERM MANAGEMENT ISSUES

Without active treatment guttate psoriasis tends to resolve within 2–3 months. One-third of patients have one episode only, another one-third go on to develop chronic plaque psoriasis, while the final one-third get episodes of guttate psoriasis with each streptococcal sore throat. In these patients a flare of guttate psoriasis may be prevented by early treatment of pharyngitis with antibiotics (e.g. penicillin V 500 mg four times per day for 7 days).

26 Guttate psoriasis. Numerous papules and small plaques are scattered widely over the back. This patient had a streptococcal sore throat 2 weeks earlier.

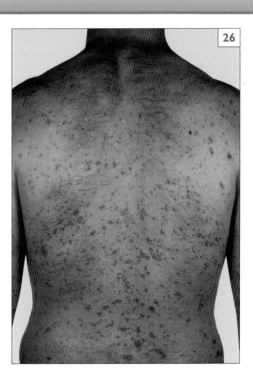

27 Guttate psoriasis. Individual lesions are deep red, slightly scaly, and measure 2–10 mm in diameter.

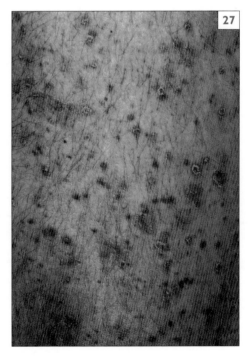

Plaque psoriasis

Active plaque psoriasis can be defined as new-onset disease or the sudden increase in numbers and size of plaques in a patient with pre-existing psoriasis. The term 'unstable' is used denote active psoriasis which has adopted an overtly inflammatory character and is rapidly expanding to produce extensive skin involvement.

CLINICAL FEATURES

In active psoriasis the lesions are red and often warm on palpation. Although scaling is often prominent (**28**) and accompanied by desquamation, in some cases unstable psoriasis may display only minimal hyperkeratosis. Occasionally pustules can be seen within very inflamed plaques of psoriasis. The usual sites are: extensor surfaces of the limbs, trunk, flexures, genitalia, scalp, and hairline (**28–32**). Actively expanding lesions can coalesce to form large plaques, especially on the torso (**28**). Itching is common and lesional skin can also be sore. Scratching of active psoriasis, especially in the scalp, can lead to secondary staphylococcal infection (**32**). Psoriasis displays the Koebner phenomenon, which is the development of lesional skin at sites of skin trauma. Nail involvement produces a dystrophy characterized by pitting, onycholysis and subungual hyperkeratosis. An acute synovitis (arthritis) may accompany active psoriatic skin involvement.

DIFFERENTIAL DIAGNOSIS

- Discoid eczema (p. 14, discrete patches of eczema, usually on lower legs).
- Seborrhoeic dermatitis (p. 20, erythema and scaling of the face, scalp and chest).
- Lichen planus (p. 36, violaceous papules and plaques, typical changes in the mouth).
- Mycosis fungoides (p. 194, pink or red patches with superficial atrophy, distributed asymmetrically).

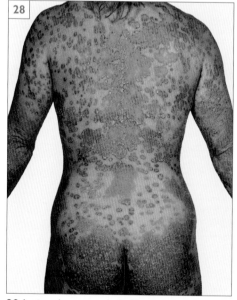

28 Active plaque psoriasis. There are numerous well demarcated, scaly plaques on the back, arms, and buttocks. These actively expanding lesions have coalesced to form large areas of involvement.

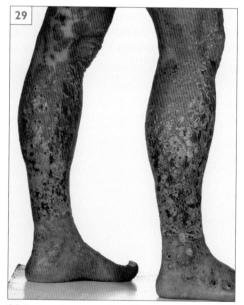

29 Active plaque psoriasis. Extensive involvement of the legs is typical in active psoriasis. The lesions are often both sore and itchy.

COMPLICATIONS
- Malaise and fatigue (with extensive involvement).
- Psoriatic arthritis.
- Erythroderma (see p. 51).

INVESTIGATIONS
- The diagnosis is usually made clinically.
- Blood count, basic chemistry, liver function tests (if considering systemic immunosuppressant therapy).
- Radiographs of affected joints.

IMMEDIATE MANAGEMENT
Topical therapy
- General emollient therapy.

- Corticosteroid ointment, twice per day (use for a restricted period):
   - face and flexures: mild.
   - trunk and limbs: moderately potent.
   - (A gauze bodysuit can be used to maximize the effects of topical therapy.)
- UVB phototherapy and psoralen-UVA (PUVA) photochemotherapy should be used carefully since these modalities can aggravate unstable psoriasis.
- Specific antipsoriatic topical agents, such as dithranol (anthralin), tend to irritate acute psoriasis and should probably be avoided at first.

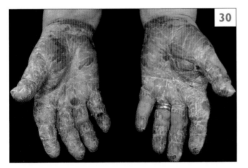

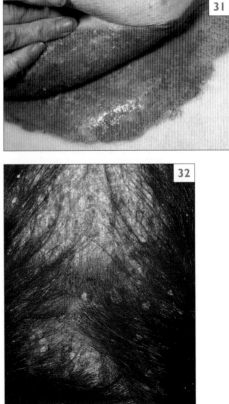

30 Palmar psoriasis. Severe, symmetrical, and confluent inflammation with hyperkeratosis of the palms. Palmar and plantar involvement is often functionally disabling. Note the sharp line of delineation at the wrists, typical for psoriasis.

31 Flexural psoriasis. In flexural skin, psoriasis is nonscaly and clearly delineated.

32 Scalp psoriasis. There is erythema and hyperkeratosis of the scalp with scale caught up in the hair. Signs of secondary bacterial infection (impetiginization) are present.

Systemic therapy

- In extensive, unstable plaque psoriasis consider treating with ciclosporin (3–5 mg/kg/day in two divided doses) or methotrexate (5 mg first dose, second dose in 7 days, thereafter 5–20 mg once per week).
- For secondary bacterial infection give oral antibiotics (e.g. flucloxacillin 500 mg four times per day for 7 days).
- A sedating oral antihistamine at bedtime will relieve itch and improve sleep (e.g. hydroxyzine 25 or 50 mg).
- A nonsteroidal anti-inflammatory drug (NSAID) for active arthritis.

LONG-TERM MANAGEMENT ISSUES

Once the psoriasis is less acutely inflamed it may respond to specific antipsoriasis topical therapies such as dithranol (anthralin), tar or vitamin D analogues. UVB phototherapy or PUVA can be used in widespread disease. If the patient is failing to respond to first- and second-line treatments or there is significant concomitant psoriatic arthritis then a systemic agent may be required, e.g. methotrexate, acitretin or ciclosporin. Biologic agents, such as etanercept, infliximab, or adalimumab, may be indicated in widespread, active psoriasis particularly if other systemic agents are found to be ineffective or poorly tolerated. Patients with moderate–severe psoriasis need to be under the care of a dermatologist. Active psoriasis may be associated with alcohol misuse and HIV infection in some cases.

Palmo-plantar pustulosis

Palmo-plantar pustulosis (PPP) is a localized form of psoriasis characterized by the development of sterile pustules on palms and soles. It usually occurs in the 5th and 6th decades with a female preponderance. Cigarette smoking is probably a provoking factor. The patient is systemically well but the condition can have a profound effect on normal daily activities.

CLINICAL FEATURES

There are well demarcated areas of erythema studded with pustules which tend to occur symmetrically on palms and/or soles (**33**). The eruption usually commences on the thenar eminences of the palms (**34**) and the instep or lateral borders of the soles, and can thereafter spread to involve all the palmo-plantar skin. Lesional skin is often scaly as well as pustular. The pustules are initially pale yellow but as they evolve become yellow–brown and then dark brown in colour. Commonly pustules in all stages of evolution are seen. Desquamation occurs as the pustules resolve (**35**). The eruption is both itchy and painful.

DIFFERENTIAL DIAGNOSIS

- Pompholyx eczema (p. 12, vesicular eczema on palmo-plantar skin).
- Tinea manum/tinea pedis (p. 154, palmar or plantar erythema and scaling, usually asymmetrical).

COMPLICATIONS

- Erysipelas/cellulitis (rare).

INVESTIGATIONS

- The diagnosis is usually made clinically.
- Skin swabs for microbiology (to exclude bacterial infection).
- Skin scrapings for mycology (to exclude dermatophyte infection).

IMMEDIATE MANAGEMENT
Topical therapy
- General emollient therapy.
- Potassium permanganate soaks once daily, following rupture of the pustules.
- Corticosteroid ointment, twice per day (use for a restricted period):
    palms and soles: potent or superpotent. (Corticosteroid efficacy can be enhanced by occlusion using polythene gloves for the hands and plastic kitchen wrap for the feet.)

LONG-TERM MANAGEMENT ISSUES
PPP tends to run a chronic course. In acute exacerbations, reintroduction of the above management plan is helpful to control pustulation. Patients with recalcitrant PPP may respond to methotrexate, ciclosporin, acitretin, or local PUVA. Biologic agents, such as etanercept, infliximab, or adalimumab, may be considered in intractable, disabling PPP. Patients with PPP need to be under the care of a dermatologist.

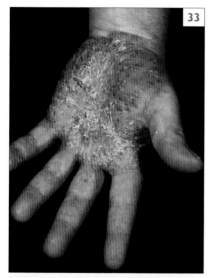

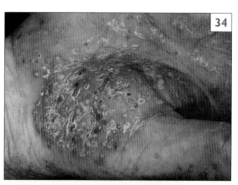

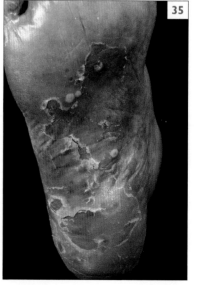

33 Palmo-plantar pustulosis. There are numerous creamy white pustules on a background of erythema. The older lesions are red–brown. Identical changes were present on the other palm.

34 Palmo-plantar pustulosis. Pustules in all stages can be seen clearly on the thenar eminence. The pustules are sterile.

35 Palmo-plantar pustulosis. In this case a few large pustules are present on the plantar arch and heel, accompanied by desquamation.

Generalized pustular psoriasis

Generalized pustular psoriasis (GPP) is the most severe form of acute psoriasis. As with palmo-plantar pustulosis, the pustules are sterile. GPP can occur in an individual with previously stable psoriasis or, less commonly, as a first presentation of psoriasis. It can be precipitated by pregnancy (**36**), the rapid withdrawal of systemic corticosteroids, an episode of sunburn, or the inappropriate use of topical dithranol and tar preparations. A patient with GPP is usually extremely ill.

CLINICAL FEATURES

The trunk, flexures, and proximal limbs are commonly involved, however in many cases patients may become erythrodermic. Affected areas are red and covered by numerous, tiny, superficial pustules (**37**). Pustules may coalesce to form large 'lakes' of pus. The intense skin inflammation is painful and often accompanied by oedema. Extension of lesional skin is characterized by periodic 'waves' of pustules which are each followed by a zone of desquamation (**38**). Secondary skin infection with *Staphylococcus aureus* can occur.

DIFFERENTIAL DIAGNOSIS

- Acute generalized exanthematous pustulosis (p. 226, a widespread pustular drug eruption).
- Subcorneal pustular dermatosis (an eruption of numerous large flaccid pustules).
- Candidiasis (p. 158, areas of flexural erythema with pustules).
- Pemphigus foliaceous (p. 68, vesicles, bullae, and scaling, especially on torso).

COMPLICATIONS

- Erythroderma (see p. 51).
- Fever.
- Malaise and weight loss.
- Hypocalcaemia.
- Liver dysfunction.
- Acute renal failure.
- Hypotension and cardiac failure.
- Deep vein thrombosis.
- Malabsorption.
- Capillary leak syndrome.
- Multiorgan failure.

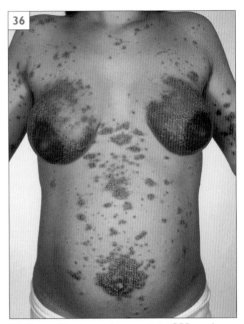

36 Generalized pustular psoriasis. GPP can be triggered by pregnancy, as with this patient. This is an extremely rare association.

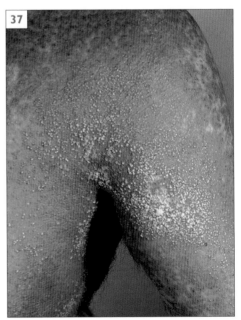

37 Generalized pustular psoriasis. There is widespread erythema with myriads of tiny pustules covering involved skin. This patient was extremely ill with a high fever and malaise.

INVESTIGATIONS
- Blood count (commonly neutrophilia and anaemia).
- Basic chemistry (renal impairment may occur).
- Liver function tests (commonly hypoalbuminaemia and elevated transaminases).
- Calcium and phosphate (serum calcium may drop suddenly).
- Erythrocyte sedimentation rate (ESR), C-reactive protein (CRP) (elevated).
- Skin swabs for microbiology (to exclude bacterial or candidal infection).
- Skin biopsy for histopathology if diagnosis is in doubt (heavy infiltrate of neutrophils in the epidermis with formation of subcorneal pustules).

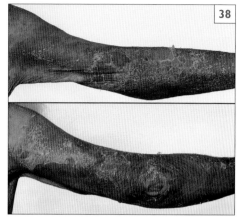

38 Generalized pustular psoriasis. Active pustulation in GPP can occur in 'waves', each of which is followed by a zone of desquamation.

IMMEDIATE MANAGEMENT
Topical therapy
- General emollient therapy.
- Corticosteroid ointment, twice per day (use for a restricted period):
    trunk, limbs: moderately potent. (The application of a topical corticosteroid is controversial since steroids can trigger pustular psoriasis; nonetheless, a moderately potent steroid ointment used initially can be a helpful therapeutic adjunct.)

Systemic therapy
- EITHER methotrexate 5 mg one dose, second dose in 5–7 days.
- OR ciclosporin 3–5 mg/kg/day in two divided doses.
- OR a biologic agent (e.g. infliximab IV infusion 5 mg/kg over 2–3 hr).
- Acitretin 25 mg once daily can control GPP (acitretin has a relatively delayed onset of action and therefore other drugs should be considered initially).

Supportive therapy
Patients with GPP should be admitted to hospital for the following:
- Bed rest and intensive topical therapy (see above).
- Monitoring of vital signs (pulse rate, blood pressure, temperature).
- Monitoring of fluid balance and administration of intravenous fluids (if required).
- Initiation of systemic therapy (see above).
- Analgesia.

LONG-TERM MANAGEMENT ISSUES
Most patients need long-term systemic therapy to maintain a remission: methotrexate, ciclosporin, acitretin, hydroxyurea, or a combination therapy (e.g. methotrexate + ciclosporin). Biologic agents, such as etanercept, infliximab, or adalimumab, may be indicated in GPP, particularly if other systemic agents are found to be ineffective or poorly tolerated. Patients with GPP need to managed by a dermatologist.

CHAPTER 3

Papular and papulo-squamous dermatoses

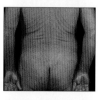 Lichen
planus

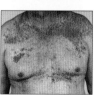 Eruptive
xanthomata

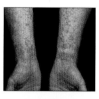 Pityriasis
rosea

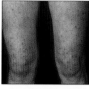 Sarcoidosis

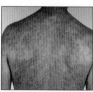 Pityriasis
rubra pilaris

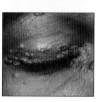 Darier's
disease

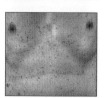 Pityriasis
lichenoides
acuta

Grover's
disease

Lichen planus

Lichen planus (LP) is a distinctive dermatosis of skin and mucous membranes. It can be localized or widespread and tends to run a prolonged course. Rarely, LP may be associated with hepatitis B and C. Although the onset may be insidious, LP not uncommonly presents as a widespread eruption of sudden onset.

CLINICAL FEATURES

The lesions of LP are shiny, flat-topped, violaceous (blue–red) papules (**39, 40**). They are often found in groups on the flexural aspects of the wrists (**40**), at the ankles (**41**), and on the low back (**42**), however any body site can be affected and lesions can be widely disseminated. The eruption is generally very itchy. Characteristic white lines cover the surface of LP lesions which are known as Wickham's striae. With time the papules may enlarge to produce plaques, nodules, or annular lesions. Blistering may occur in very inflammatory LP. The oral mucosa is commonly involved with a white, lace-like pattern on the buccal mucosae (**43**). Nails can also be involved, with features ranging from longitudinal white lines to scarring and loss of nail plates. Scalp involvement is less common but can result in scarring alopecia (lichen plano-pilaris). LP exhibits the Koebner phenomenon (**40**).

DIFFERENTIAL DIAGNOSIS

- Plaque psoriasis (p. 28, scaly plaques in symmetrical distribution with typical nail changes).
- Guttate psoriasis (p. 26, multiple, tiny, scaly papules scattered over the torso and limbs).
- Pityriasis rosea (p. 38, an eruption of slightly scaly patches following an initial 'herald' lesion).
- Secondary syphilis (p. 136, papulo-squamous eruption with acral involvement).
- Sarcoidosis (p. 46, nonscaly violaceous papules and plaques).
- Lichenoid drug eruption (papulo-squamous drug eruption).

COMPLICATIONS

- Severe orogenital ulceration (rare).

INVESTIGATIONS

- Skin biopsy for histopathology if the diagnosis is in doubt (a band-like lymphocytic infiltrate at the dermoepidermal junction causing 'saw-tooth' effacement of the rete ridges; apoptotic keratinocytes are seen in the basal layer of the epidermis).
- Liver function tests (if hepatitis is suspected).
- Hepatitis B and C serology (if hepatitis is suspected).

IMMEDIATE MANAGEMENT
Topical therapy
- General emollient therapy.
- Corticosteroid ointment, twice per day (use for a restricted period):
    trunk and limbs: potent or superpotent.
- A steroid mouthwash for oral symptoms.

Systemic therapy
- A sedating oral antihistamine at bedtime (e.g. hydroxyzine 25 or 50 mg) will relieve itch and improve sleep.
- In widespread LP a short, reducing course of oral corticosteroid can control the eruption and relieve pruritus (e.g. prednisolone 20–30 mg for 5 days and reduce by 5 mg each week).

LONG-TERM MANAGEMENT ISSUES

LP is often long-lasting, tending to resolve within 12–18 months. The papules and plaques flatten usually leaving postinflammatory hyper-pigmentation which can be prominent and persistent in pigmented skin. If oral ulceration is present and severe then an oral immunosuppressant (e.g. ciclosporin) may be required. Widespread, recalcitrant skin involve-ment can be treated with a course of phototherapy (UVB, PUVA) or with a systemic medication (e.g. ciclosporin, azathioprine). LP of the scalp can result in scarring alopecia, while nail involvement can lead to irreversible scarring of the nail bed, therefore, in these situations, the prompt introduction of systemic immunosuppressant therapy may be necessary.

39 Lichen planus. In acute LP there is an eruption of violaceous papules. The inner aspects of the wrists and forearms are common sites of involvement.

40 Lichen planus. The individual lesions of LP are flat-topped and shiny. The eruption is usually itchy and displays Koebner's phenomenon in which lesions develop at sites of sctratching (as shown).

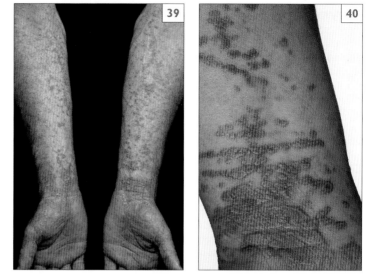

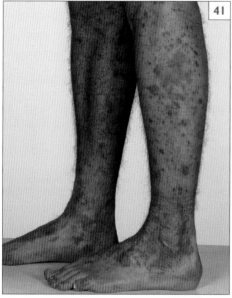

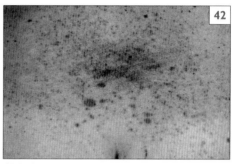

42 Lichen planus. Lesions can be widely disseminated over the body.

41 Lichen planus. The lower legs and ankles are often involved.

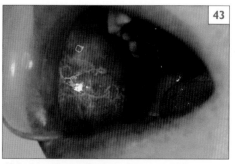

43 Lichen planus. Oral involvement in LP is common and usually produces a network of white lines on the buccal mucosae. Lichenoid changes may also occur on the lips, tongue, gingivae, and palate.

Pityriasis rosea

Pityriasis rosea (PR) is a common acute eruption which generally affects young adults and children. It is thought to represent a viral exanthem; studies have implicated the involvement of human herpesvirus 6 (HHV6) or HHV7. The eruption of PR usually has a sudden onset and is often widespread causing patients to present acutely.

CLINICAL FEATURES

The first clinical sign is a solitary 'herald' patch usually on the torso or on a thigh or upper arm. It can reach sizes of 2–5 cm in diameter and is well demarcated, inflamed and covered by a fine scale (**44**). Seven to 14 days later a widespread eruption occurs on the torso and proximal limbs consisting of numerous, red, oval patches (**45, 46**). These lesions tend to follow Langer's lines to produce a 'Christmas tree' pattern on the back. They often have a surface scale that peels from the centre leaving a collarette of scale. The eruption may be itchy but is commonly asymptomatic. Some patients, particularly those with pigmented skins, produce overtly eczematous lesions (**47**). In occasional cases the lesions will have a predilection for the limbs and flexures, instead of the trunk, and is known as PR inversus.

DIFFERENTIAL DIAGNOSIS

- Guttate psoriasis (p. 26, multiple, tiny, scaly papules scattered over the torso and limbs).
- Plaque psoriasis (p. 28, scaly plaques in symmetrical distribution with typical nail changes).
- Tinea corporis (p. 154, scaly, annular, inflammatory patches distributed asymmetrically).
- Secondary syphilis (p. 136, papulo-squamous eruption with acral involvement).

COMPLICATIONS

- Flu-like symptoms (occasional).

INVESTIGATIONS

- The diagnosis is usually made clinically.
- Skin scrapings for mycology (if a dermatophyte infection is suspected).
- Skin biopsy for histopathology if the diagnosis is in doubt (epidermal undulation, focal spongiosis with lymphocytic exocytosis).

IMMEDIATE MANAGEMENT

Many cases will not require active treatment.

Topical therapy

- General emollient therapy.
- Corticosteroid ointment, twice per day (use for a restricted period):
    trunk and limbs: moderately potent.

Systemic therapy

- There is some evidence that high-dose oral aciclovir can accelerate resolution (800 mg 5 times per day for 1 week).

LONG-TERM MANAGEMENT ISSUES

PR will usually resolve within 6 weeks. UVB phototherapy can be considered for more resistant cases.

44 Pityriasis rosea. The herald patch is the first lesion to appear and remains larger than the other patches of PR. The herald patch often displays a collarette of scale.

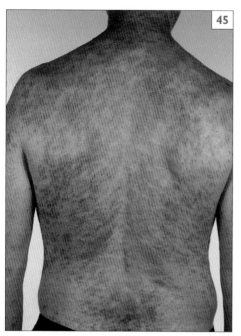

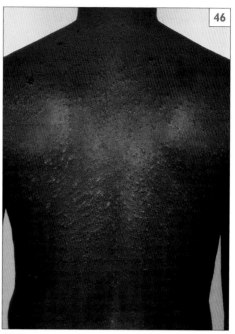

45 Pityriasis rosea. There are numerous, oval, pink patches on the torso. The lesions align themselves along Langer's lines. The body and proximal limbs are usually maximally involved.

46 Pityriasis rosea. In dark skin the lesions are often hyperpigmented.

47 Pityriasis rosea. In some patients, especially individuals with pigmented skin, PR can produce lesions which are raised, inflammatory, and look eczematous or lichenoid.

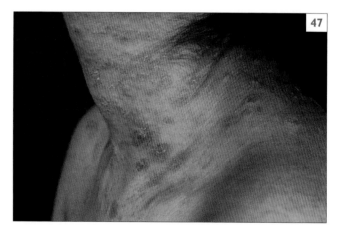

Pityriasis rubra pilaris

Pityriasis rubra pilaris (PRP) is a rare, papulo-squamous dermatosis of unknown aetiology. In the adult form it usually progresses rapidly to become widespread and highly symptomatic.

CLINICAL FEATURES
The earliest signs are inflammation and hyperkeratosis of the skin's hair follicles producing an eruption of rough, red papules. These papules coalesce to produce large areas of orange–red erythema within which are zones of unaffected skin, so-called 'islands of sparing' (**48**). The eruption is often itchy and can also be sore. PRP usually starts on the head and then spreads caudally to involve the torso, arms, and, finally, the legs. Erythrodermic involvement can occur rapidly and may be accompanied by a range of constitutional symptoms associated with total skin inflammation (see Chapter 4) (**49**). Palmo-plantar involvement produces a thick orange–yellow hyperkeratosis (keratoderma) (**49**). Involvement of the nails is characterized by subungual hyperkeratosis, dystrophy, and splinter haemorrhages.

DIFFERENTIAL DIAGNOSIS
- Any cause of erythroderma (p. 51, complete, confluent skin involvement by any dermatosis).
- Plaque psoriasis (p. 28, scaly plaques in symmetrical distribution with typical nail changes).
- Seborrhoeic dermatitis (p. 20, erythema and scaling of the face, scalp, and chest).

COMPLICATIONS
- Erythroderma (see p. 51).

INVESTIGATIONS
- Blood count, basic chemistry, liver function tests (needed if considering systemic immunosuppressant therapy or patient systemically unwell).
- Skin biopsy for histopathology (follicles are dilated, filled with keratin, and show perifollicular parakeratosis; there is hypergranulosis of the interfollicular epidermis and a lymphohistiocytic perivascular infiltrate in the dermis).

IMMEDIATE MANAGEMENT
Topical therapy
- General emollient therapy.
- Corticosteroid ointment, twice per day (use for a restricted period):
    face: mildly potent.
    trunk and limbs: moderately potent.

Systemic therapy
- Sedating and nonsedating antihistamines.
- Acitretin (20–30 mg daily) or isotretinoin (0.5–1.0 mg/kg daily).
- Methotrexate (10–20 mg once per week).

LONG-TERM MANAGEMENT ISSUES
The classical adult form of PRP is a chronic dermatosis but usually self-limiting, typically clearing within 3 years in 80% of patients. During this period patients require regular assessments from a dermatologist and treatment with acitretin or methotrexate which can modify the disease and, in some cases, can clear the eruption. Biologic agents, such as etanercept, infliximab, or adalimumab, may be indicated in PRP, particularly if other systemic agents are found to be ineffective or poorly tolerated.

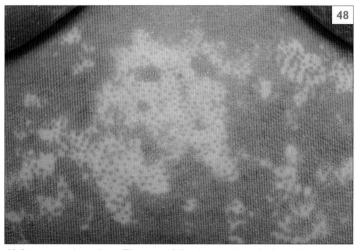

48 Pityriasis rubra pilaris. There are follicular papules which coalesce to form large areas of erythema. Within zones of lesional skin there are islands of sparing; this sign is typical for PRP.

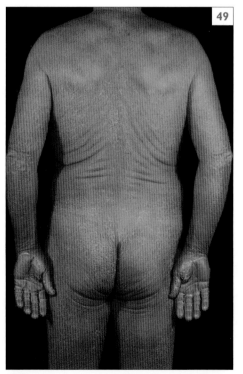

49 Pityriasis rubra pilaris. PRP often extends rapidly to cause erythroderma. It is associated with scaling and thick hyperkeratosis of the palms and soles.

Pityriasis lichenoides acuta

Pityriasis lichenoides acuta (or pityriasis lichenoides et varioliformis acuta) is a rare, cutaneous T cell lymphoproliferative disorder. Although there is lymphocyte clonality, it is not a cutaneous lymphoma. The chronic form of pityriasis lichenoides is a relatively indolent dermatosis, whereas the acute disease presents with striking skin signs and usually prompts the patient to seek an urgent opinion.

CLINICAL FEATURES

Multiple small papules and vesicles appear in crops on any skin site, mostly the limbs. The lesions tend to develop in a polymorphic manner (**50**); some are scaly, others evolve into small necrotic ulcers which may become infected or heal with scarring (**51**). The skin lesions are generally not itchy, but may be painful, and tend to resolve spontaneously within a few weeks. Onset of the eruption is sometimes accompanied by constitutional symptoms.

DIFFERENTIAL DIAGNOSIS

- Small vessel vasculitis (p. 82, multiple, palpable, purpuric lesions, usually on the lower legs).
- Guttate psoriasis (p. 26, multiple, tiny, scaly papules scattered over the torso and limbs).
- Lymphomatoid papulosis (a lympho-proliferative disorder of red papules which become necrotic).

COMPLICATIONS

- Fever and malaise.
- Lymphadenopathy.
- Arthralgia.

INVESTIGATIONS

Skin biopsy is performed for histopathology (interface and upper dermal wedge-shaped lymphocytic infiltrate with erythrocyte extravasation and, in advanced lesions, epidermal necrosis).

IMMEDIATE MANAGEMENT
Topical therapy

- General emollient therapy.
- Corticosteroid ointment, twice per day (use for a restricted period):
    trunk and limbs: moderately potent or potent.

Systemic therapy

- In severe and extensive pityriasis lichenoides acuta a short, reducing course of oral corticosteroids can be helpful in inducing a remission (e.g. prednisolone 20–30 mg/day for 5 days and reducing by 5 mg each week).
- A short course of erythromycin is often beneficial (500 mg four times per day for 2 weeks).

LONG-TERM MANAGEMENT ISSUES

The eruption tends to resolve spontaneously within a few weeks. Healing of necrotic lesions may occur with scarring. The chronic form of pityriasis lichenoides is a relapsing–remitting dermatosis characterized by red–brown papules and plaques which often have an overlying scale. These lesions tend to persist for many weeks or months before resolving to leave hypopigmented macules.

50 Pityriasis lichenoides acuta. The eruption is polymorphic; in this case there are red papules, some of which are scaly, and necrotic lesions.

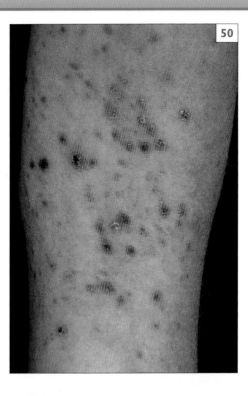

51 Pityriasis lichenoides acuta. This patient with extensive involvement shows numerous necrotic lesions on the legs, some having healed with scarring.

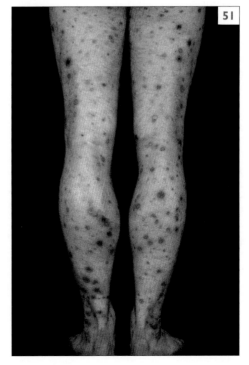

Eruptive xanthomata

Xanthomata are cutaneous deposits of lipid which appear in a variety of forms and occur, in most cases, as a manifestation of hyperlipidaemia. It is important to recognize xanthomata since the associated metabolic anomalies are linked to accelerated atherosclerosis. The eruptive form of xanthoma represents a distinctive clinical pattern which, as the name suggests, develops suddenly and is associated with certain types of lipid dysfunction.

CLINICAL FEATURES

Eruptive xanthomata appear rapidly over pressure points and on extensor surfaces, especially elbows, knees, and buttocks (**52**). The eruption is monomorphic (the lesions all look the same) and is comprised of discrete papules measuring 1–3 mm in diameter. Clinically, the lesions have a characteristic yellow colour and appear waxy (**53**). They are sometimes umbilicated and may possess a red halo.

DIFFERENTIAL DIAGNOSIS

- Molluscum contagiosum (a pox virus infection causing skin-coloured umbilicated papules).
- Folliculitis (p. 120, bacterial infection of hair follicles causing papules and pustules).
- Xanthoma disseminatum (a histiocytosis of flexural xanthomatous papules with diabetes insipidus).

COMPLICATIONS

- Accelerated atherosclerosis.

INVESTIGATIONS

- Lipid profile (the lipid abnormalities will reflect the type of hyperlipidaemia).
- Blood glucose, liver function tests, thyroid function tests.
- Skin biopsy for histopathology (an aggregate of foamy histiocytes and multinucleated giant cells in the dermis).

IMMEDIATE MANAGEMENT

Treat the underlying lipid disorder with dietary modification and lipid-lowering drugs.

LONG-TERM MANAGEMENT ISSUES

The patient must be referred to an internal physician for appropriate evaluation and assessment of other cardiovascular risk factors. Eruptive xanthomata occur in familial dysbetalipoproteinaemia, familial lipoprotein lipase deficiency, and familial hypertriglyceridaemia. Other medical conditions associated with secondary hyperlipidaemia, complicated by eruptive xanthomata include nephrotic syndrome, hypothyroidism, monoclonal gammopathies, and alcoholism. Drug-induced hyperlipoproteinaemia has also been implicated in contributing to the formation of eruptive xanthomata; culprit drugs include oestrogens, corticosteroids, and retinoids.

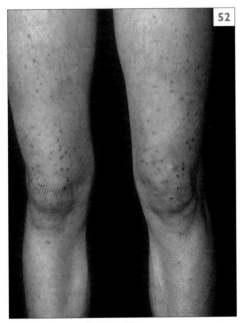

52 Eruptive xanthomata. There are numerous papules and nodules on the knees and anterior thighs. Extensor surfaces are a common site for eruptive xanthomata.

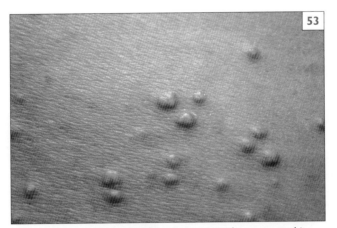

53 Eruptive xanthomata. Close inspection reveals monomorphic, smooth papules which are a pale yellow colour.

Sarcoidosis

Sarcoidosis is a multisystem disease of granulomatous inflammation. The lymph nodes, lungs, liver, eyes, and skin are most frequently involved and it is not uncommon for sarcoidosis to present with cutaneous manifestations. Skin sarcoid usually runs a chronic course, however some cases present acutely with the sudden onset of highly visible skin lesions and associated systemic features.

CLINICAL FEATURES
There is a wide range of lesion type in cutaneous sarcoidosis, however papules (often tiny) and plaques are seen most commonly. Lesions are usually smooth-surfaced and asymptomatic. The colour may be brownish or violaceous (blue–red). Involvement of the face is typical, occurring particularly around the eyes (**54**) and on the nasal alae. Skin sarcoid can also present as plaques (**55**), nodules, annular lesions, hypopigmented patches (in dark skin), and scarring alopecia. Lupus pernio is an infiltrative form of cutaneous sarcoid characterized by violaceous plaques on the nasal tip (**56**), cheeks, and ears. Sarcoid in the skin and deeper tissue of a finger can result in dactylitis (**57**). Sarcoid can also present with erythema nodosum (see p. 100).

DIFFERENTIAL DIAGNOSIS
- Discoid lupus erythematosus (p. 106, well demarcated plaques of scarring erythema, especially on the face).
- Lichen planus (p. 36, violaceous papules and plaques with typical changes in the mouth).
- Syringomata (benign sweat gland tumours, usually multiple, occurring as papules on the eyelids).
- Acne agminata (a papular facial eruption of granulomatous inflammation).
- Cutaneous tuberculosis (lupus vulgaris) (infiltrating, scarring plaques of tuberculosis occurring on the face).

COMPLICATIONS
- Malaise and weight loss.
- Lymphadenopathy.
- Pulmonary involvement (upper airway involvement, hilar lymphadenopathy, interstial infiltration/fibrosis).
- Neurological involvement (peipheral and central nervous system disorders).
- Ocular involvement (especially uveitis).
- Hepatic involvement.
- Cardiac involvement.

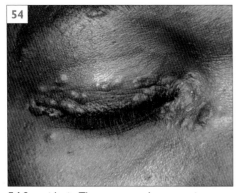

54 Sarcoidosis. There are papules occurring on the eyelids and around the eyes. This is a typical site for cutaneous sarcoidosis.

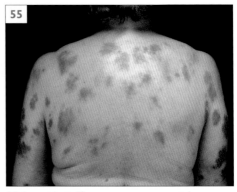

55 Sarcoidosis. There are numerous violaceous plaques on the back of this patient who also had pulmonary and ocular sarcoidosis.

INVESTIGATIONS
- Blood count, routine chemistry, liver function tests (raised transaminases in hepatic sarcoid).
- ESR (elevated in active sarcoidosis).
- Calcium and phosphate (hypercalcaemia).
- Serum angiotensin-3 converting enzyme (ACE) (elevated in extensive sarcoidosis).
- Chest radiography (bilateral hilar lymphadenopathy, pulmonary infiltration, and fibrosis).
- High resolution computed tomography (CT) scan of chest (bilateral hilar lymphadenopathy, pulmonary infiltration, and fibrosis).
- Pulmonary function tests (restrictive defect).
- Electrocardiogram (ECG) (to exclude cardiac involvement).
- Skin biopsy for histopathology (granulomatous infiltrate in the upper dermis composed of lymphocyte-poor granulomas).

IMMEDIATE MANAGEMENT
Topical therapy
- Corticosteroid ointment, twice per day (use for a restricted period):
  - face: moderately potent or potent.
  - trunk and limbs: potent or superpotent.
- Intralesional triamcinolone injections.
- Tacrolimus ointment.

Systemic therapy
- In widespread skin sarcoid or symptomatic systemic involvement, oral corticosteroid may be given (e.g. prednisolone 20–30 mg/day and reducing with response).

LONG-TERM MANAGEMENT ISSUES
Oral corticosteroids are the mainstay treatment in many cases and, if required over a long period, should be tapered to a low maintenance dose. Prolonged use of systemic corticosteroids requires an on-going screening programme for diabetes, hypertension, and osteoporosis. Osteoporosis prophylaxis is recommended. Azathioprine can be used as a steroid-sparing agent. Methotrexate can also be used with good efficacy in some patients. Hydroxychloroquine (100–200 mg twice per day, or 6.5 mg/kg/day) and other antimalarials can be effective in some cases. The anti-tumour necrosis factor (TNF) biological agents infliximab and adalimumab have been used with success in severe sarcoidosis. Localized papules and plaques of sarcoid on the face can respond to laser ablation. Cosmetic camouflage make-up can be extremely helpful in disfiguring facial sarcoid. Patients with cutaneous sarcoidosis must be under the care of a dermatologist, systemic involvement requires management by an internal physician.

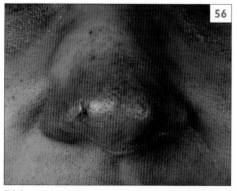

56 Sarcoidosis. Lupus pernio is characterized by diffuse, violaceous infiltration of the nasal tip.

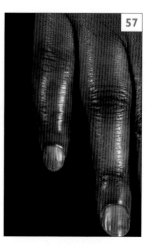

57 Sarcoidosis. Sarcoid dactylitis causes painful, deep swelling of affected digits.

Darier's disease

Darier's disease is a rare genodermatosis affecting the ATP2A2 gene causing defects in intracellular calcium signalling. It is inherited in an autosomal dominant pattern with variable expression. Most patients present with skin problems in puberty. The disease course is chronic but is often punctuated by episodic acute flares. Darier's disease can be aggravated by UV radiation (strong sunshine) or by secondary bacterial or viral skin infection.

CLINICAL FEATURES

There are red–brown scaly papules (**58**) found principally on the face, scalp, neck, central chest, and back. Individual lesions may coalesce to form scaly patches which are often itchy (**59**). Flexural involvement is common and can lead to macerated, malodorous plaques in the axillae and groins. Nail involvement produces alternating pink and white longitudinal lines and V-shaped notching of the free margin. Examination of the mouth may reveal cobble-stone papules on the palate. Secondary infection of lesional skin in Darier's disease will cause an inflammatory flare which leads to worsening itch and soreness (**59**). HSV infection causes erosions and haemorrhagic crusts while *Staphylococcus aureus* colonization produces yellow–brown crusting (**60**).

DIFFERENTIAL DIAGNOSIS

- Seborrhoeic dermatitis (p. 20, erythema and scaling of the face, scalp, and chest).
- Grover's disease (p. 50, keratotic papules on torso of sun-damaged patients).
- Hailey Hailey disease (red–brown scaly papules, predominantly in flexures).

COMPLICATIONS

- Malaise and fatigue (with extensive involvement).
- Secondary bacterial or herpetic infection.
- Regional lymphadenopathy (with secondary infection).
- Fever (with severe secondary infection).

INVESTIGATIONS

- Skin biopsy for histopathology (suprabasal acantholysis and dyskeratosis).
- Skin swab for bacteriology (if secondary bacterial infection is suspected).
- Skin swab for virology (if secondary viral infection is suspected).
- Serum lipids, liver function tests (if oral retinoids are being considered).

IMMEDIATE MANAGEMENT
Topical therapy

- General emollient therapy.
- Corticosteroid ointment, twice per day (use for a restricted period):
    face: mildly potent.
    trunk and limbs: potent.
- High protection factor sunscreen.

Systemic therapy

- A sedating oral antihistamine at bedtime will relieve itch (e.g. hydroxyzine 25 or 50 mg).
- For suspected HSV infection: oral aciclovir 200 mg five times per day for 5 days.
- For suspected *S. aureus* infection: oral flucloxacillin 500 mg four times per day for 7 days.

LONG-TERM MANAGEMENT ISSUES

Patients with Darier's disease need to be considered for oral retinoid therapy, e.g. acitretin or etretinate, which, when taken over a prolonged period, can reduce frequency of inflammatory flares. Regular follow-up by a dermatologist is important to monitor long-term therapy and to manage acute relapses. Some patients suffer from a variety of neuropsychiatric problems, including epilepsy, learning difficulties, and shizo-affective disorder.

58 Darier's disease. The individual lesions of Darier's disease are red–brown papules with a roughened, often crusted, surface.

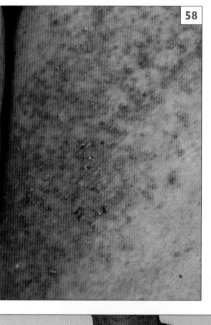

59 Darier's disease. There is an eruption of keratotic papules on the torso which have become confluent in areas. Features suggesting secondary infection with S. *aureus* are seen on the chest.

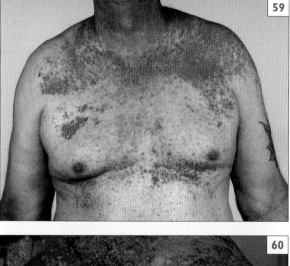

60 Darier's disease. This patient has developed a grossly hyperkeratotic and fissured area on the back which is secondarily infected. The involved skin is malodorous.

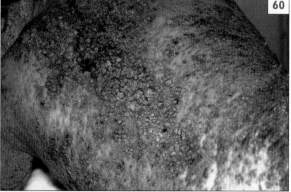

Grover's disease

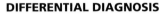

Grover's disease is an unusual papulo-squamous eruption on the torso, probably caused by an excessive cumulative exposure to UV radiation. As well as sunlight, acute flares can be triggered by heat and sweating.

CLINICAL FEATURES

The typical patient is a middle-aged man with sun-damaged skin. There is an eruption of multiple pink papules or papulo-vesicles on the chest and back (**61**). The eruption is itchy and the papules become crusted with time (**62**).

DIFFERENTIAL DIAGNOSIS

- Miliaria (p. 204, monomorphic red papules on the torso and flexures).
- Solar keratoses (intraepidermal dysplasia: multiple, small, scaly, red patches on exposed skin).
- Seborrhoeic dermatitis (p. 20, erythema and scaling of the face, scalp, and chest).
- Darier's disease (p. 48, red–brown scaly papules on face, neck, chest, and flexures).

COMPLICATIONS

There are usually none.

INVESTIGATIONS

Skin biopsy is performed for histopathology (clefting within the epidermis with focal areas of acantholysis and dyskeratosis).

IMMEDIATE MANAGEMENT
Topical therapy

- General emollient therapy.
- Corticosteroid ointment, twice per day (use for a restricted period):
    trunk and limbs: potent.
- High protection factor sunscreen.

LONG-TERM MANAGEMENT ISSUES

Grover's disease can run a self-limiting course but in some patients may be persistent. Patients with recalcitrant disease might respond to oral retinoid therapy, e.g. acitretin or etretinate, although this is not effective in every case. All patients with Grover's disease should receive photoprotection advice.

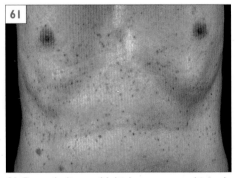

61 Grover's disease. Multiple, monomorphic red papules on the torso. Typically Grover's disease is itchy.

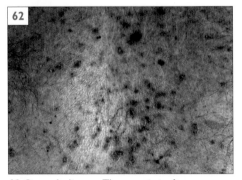

62 Grover's disease. The eruption often occurs on photodamaged skin. The lesions can be scaly and crusted.

CHAPTER 4

Erythroderma

Erythroderma is a descriptive term which refers to any skin disease involving greater than 80–90% of the body surface area. Patients may develop erythroderma as a first presentation of a skin disorder or following uncontrolled activity of a pre-existing dermatosis. Since an adverse drug reaction can result in erythroderma it is important to obtain a detailed drug history in all patients. Involvement of the whole skin surface interferes with a range of homeostatic mechanisms and produces constitutional as well as cutaneous clinical features. The clinical approach to a patient with erythroderma should therefore be directed to: (1) identifying the cause; (2) initiating specific therapy for the primary skin pathology; (3) addressing the systemic complications of total skin inflammation.

CLINICAL FEATURES

There is confluent erythema (>80–90% body surface area) often with scaling and desquamation (exfoliative dermatitis) (**63**). In many cases pruritus is intense (especially in Sézary syndrome); other features common to all cases of erythroderma include palmo-plantar hyperkeratosis, diffuse nonscarring alopecia, nail dystrophy, and mild generalized lymphadenopathy (dermatopathic). Although the physical signs can be relatively uniform, various clinical features may help to discriminate the different causes of erythroderma, e.g characteristic nail changes in psoriasis (pitting, onycholysis, subungual hyperkeratosis), marked lymphadenopathy in Sézary syndrome, follicular prominence and islands of sparing in PRP. The systemic sequelae to erythroderma vary between patients: in some cases the extent and degree of inflammation produce a severe illness with fever, shivering and prostration, whereas in others the erythrodermic state is relatively well tolerated.

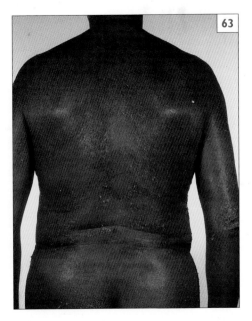

63 Erythrodermic eczema. There is confluent erythema and scaling in this patient with longstanding, poorly controlled eczema.

CAUSES OF ERYTHRODERMA

Any dermatosis, if extensive, can cause erythroderma.

- Plaque psoriasis (p. 28, confluent scaly plaques, nail changes).
- Generalized pustular psoriasis (p.32, widespread erythema with myriads of tiny pustules) (**64**).
- Atopic dermatitis (p. 8, eczema as part of atopic diathesis).
- Seborrhoeic dermatitis (p. 20, exaggerated involvement of scalp, face, and flexures).
- Systematized allergic contact/chronic actinic dermatitis (pp. 18, 22, history of eczema initially in a localized area).
- Drug reactions (pp. 220, 224, 226, 230, a variety of reaction patterns following medication exposure) (**65**).
- Mycosis fungoides (p. 194, T cell lymphoma with confluent patches, plaques, and tumours).
- Sézary syndrome (p. 194, T cell lymphoma with confluent erythema and marked lymphadenopathy).
- Pityriasis rubra pilaris (p. 40, confluent erythema with follicular prominence and islands of sparing).
- Pemphigoid/pemphigus (pp. 66, 68, widespread erythema with blisters and erosions).
- Graft-versus-host disease (p. 218, widespread erythema following haematopoietic allogeneic stem cell transplantation).
- Paraneoplastic erythroderma (widespread erythema associated with underlying tumour).

COMPLICATIONS

- Fever, malaise, fatigue.
- Hypo- and hyperthermia.
- Weight loss and malabsorption.
- Lymphadenopathy.
- Secondary bacterial infection leading to systemic sepsis.
- Tachycardia, hypotension, and cardiac failure.
- Acute renal failure.
- Liver dysfunction.
- Thromboembolic disease.
- Capillary leak syndrome.

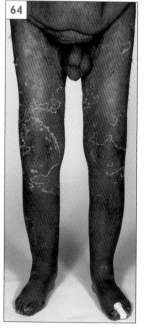

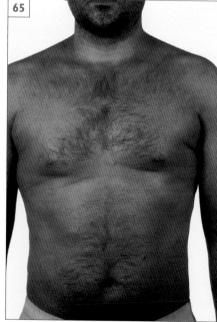

64 Erythrodermic psoriasis. This patient with unstable psoriasis had recently suffered a flare of generalized pustular psoriasis. There are confluent erythema, zones of desquamation, and dependent oedema.

65 Erythrodermic drug rash. This patient with gout developed a hypersensitivity reaction to allopurinol, resulting in erythroderma.

INVESTIGATIONS

- Blood count, differential white cell count, including Sézary count (anaemia and eosinophilia is common; atypical lymphocytes are often seen and are not necessarily indicative of Sézary syndrome).
- Basic chemistry, liver function tests (hypoalbuminaemia is common).
- ESR, CRP (often raised).
- Immunoglobulins, serum protein electrophoresis (IgE is often elevated).
- Chest radiography, ECG.
- T cell receptor gene rearrangement studies on skin, blood, and lymph node (if cutaneous T cell lymphoma is suspected).
- Skin swab for microbiology (if secondary bacterial infection suspected).
- Skin biopsy for histopathology – sometimes several biopsies are needed to demonstrate useful diagnostic features. A definitive diagnosis may not be revealed in many cases of erythroderma and clinicopathological correlation is essential; psoriasiform epidermal hyperplasia and spongiosis do not necessarily indicate psoriasis and dermatitis, respectively; a chronic inflammatory cell infiltrate in the upper dermis is usual; eosinophils are not always present in drug-related cases, however an occasional apoptotic keratinocyte may indicate a drug sensitivity. See other chapters for disease-specific dermatopathology.
- Skin biopsy for direct immunofluorescence (if pemphigus or pemphigoid is suspected).
- Lymph node biopsy (if Sézary syndrome is suspected).

IMMEDIATE MANAGEMENT
Topical therapy
- General emollient therapy.
- Corticosteroid ointment, twice per day (use for a restricted period):
  face: mildly potent.
  trunk and limbs: moderately potent.
- CAUTION: large quantities of corticosteroid can be absorbed across erythrodermic skin causing adrenal suppression; topical steroids should be used with caution in erythroderma.

Systemic therapy
Usually systemic therapy is required; the choice of agent will be directed by the underlying diagnosis (see other chapters for the management of specific dermatoses).
- For secondary bacterial infection give oral antibiotics (antistaphylococcal).
- A sedating oral antihistamine at bedtime will relieve itch and improve sleep (e.g. hydroxyzine 25 or 50 mg).

Supportive therapy
Most patients with erythroderma will need admitting to hospital for the following:
- Bed rest and intensive topical therapy (see above).
- Initiation of systemic therapy.
- Monitoring of vital signs (pulse rate, blood pressure, temperature).
- Monitoring of fluid balance.
- Administration of intravenous fluids, if required.
- Maintaining a good nutritional input.
- Monitoring of body temperature regulation.

Significant systemic complications (such as renal impairment, cardiac failure) should prompt a referral to the general physicians.

LONG-TERM MANAGEMENT ISSUES
Patients with erythroderma need to be under the care of a dermatologist. Uncontrolled erythroderma is associated with systemic complications and there is a significant associated mortality which is most marked in the elderly. In cases where the diagnosis is initially unclear, a hospital admission for diagnostic tests and intensive topical therapy can usually reveal the underlying pathology. This will then direct further specific therapy. In some cases erythroderma can persist for years without a definitive diagnosis being made, however a number of these patients will ultimately go on to develop cutaneous T cell lymphoma (Sézary syndrome).

Urticaria

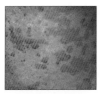 **Acute urticaria**

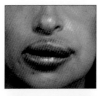 **Angio-oedema**

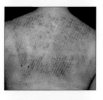 **The physical urticarias**

 Urticarial vasculitis

Acute urticaria

Acute urticaria is a common disorder. It can be either allergic (a reaction between an antigen and specific mast cell-bound IgE) or nonallergic. Recognized precipitants include drugs (commonly aspirin, NSAIDs, antibiotics, opiates), foods (e.g. shellfish, nuts, food dyes), and infections (Epstein–Barr virus, hepatitis B, *Streptococcus*). Contact urticaria occurs when an allergen is absorbed across skin or mucous membranes producing a localized or systemic reaction (e.g. latex allergy). However, in many cases a specific trigger is not identified. Acute urticaria usually presents as a widespread, extremely itchy eruption often with a sudden onset.

CLINICAL FEATURES

Typically numerous pink weals (superficial dermal swellings) develop over the trunk and limbs. Individual lesions can display a variety of shapes, including oval, annular or arcuate forms (**66**). These may coalesce to produce large, oedematous plaques with irregular outlines. Somes weals are surrounded by a red or white halo (**67**). The weals are generally extremely itchy. Each lesion persists for a few hours (always less than 24 hours) before resolving to leave normal skin. Urticaria is a dynamic disorder in which new weals develop as older lesions resolve (**68**). Patients may display positive dermographism, which is the tendency to develop linear weals at the site of gentle scratching of the skin. Acute urticaria sometimes occurs with concomitant angio-oedema and rarely as part of an anaphylaxis reaction.

DIFFERENTIAL DIAGNOSIS

- Physical urticaria (p. 60, weals provoked by physical stimulus).
- Urticarial vasculitis (p. 62, itchy and burning weals which are persistent).
- Erythema multiforme (p. 144, urticated or blistered target-like lesions especially on acral skin).
- Bullous pemphigoid, pre-bullous phase (p. 66, itchy, urticated plaques).

COMPLICATIONS

- Fatigue and headache.
- Gastrointestinal upset.
- Arthralgia.
- Anaphylaxis (bronchospasm, laryngeal oedema, hypotension, cardiac dysrhythmia).

INVESTIGATIONS

- The diagnosis is usually made clinically.
- Radioallergosorbent tests (RAST) for specific IgE (e.g. to nuts).
- Skin prick tests for IgE-mediated reactions to suspected allergens (full resuscitation facilities should be available when challenge tests are undertaken).
- Serology if an underlying infection is suspected (EBV, hepatitis B, *Streptococcus*).

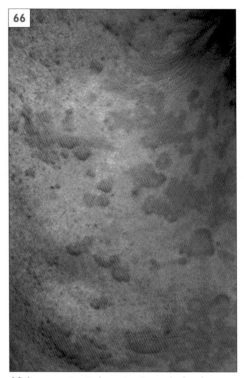

66 Acute urticaria. In urticaria weals develop with various shapes and sizes.

IMMEDIATE MANAGEMENT
Topical therapy
- Advise patient to keep skin cool (e.g. tepid baths).
- Apply a cooling emollient frequently (e.g. 1% menthol in aqueous cream).

Systemic therapy
- An H1 antihistamine is usually effective (e.g. cetirizine 10 mg or levocetirizine 5 mg once daily). Sometimes antihistamines need to be given in supranormal doses.
- A sedating antihistamine taken at bedtime can also be helpful (e.g. hydroxyzine 25–50 mg).
- In severe, widespread involvement a moderate dose of prednisolone (e.g. 20–30 mg/day) can be used for a short period (less than 2 weeks).

Supportive therapy
Treat anaphylaxis with:
- IM or SC epinephrine (adrenaline) 0.5–1.0 mg.
- Slow IV injection of chlorpheniramine 10–20 mg.
- IV hydrocortisone sodium succinate 100–300 mg.
- Oxygen.

LONG-TERM MANAGEMENT ISSUES
Chronic urticaria, which is often an auto-immune disorder, is defined as the continued development of weals for more than 6 weeks. Patients need to be under the care of a dermatologist for further investigation and second-line therapy, which may include a combination of H1 antihistamines, H2 anti-histamines, montelukast, and immunosuppressants. Patients who develop acute urticaria to a specific trigger should be encouraged to wear an appropriately marked medical alert amulet. Patients at risk of anaphylaxis should also carry an epinephrine 300 µg autoinjector (e.g. Epipen) and be able to use it appropriately.

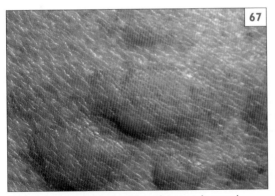

67 Acute urticaria. Urticarial weals are pink or red, oedematous, and have a smooth surface. Each weal develops and resolves within 24 hr.

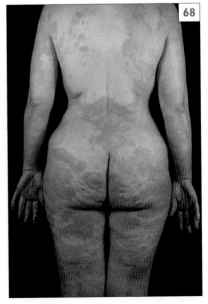

68 Acute urticaria. Involvement is often widespread. In this patient there are weals in various stages of evolution. Newer lesions, such as those on the legs, often have a pale halo.

Angio-oedema

Angio-oedema is a variant of urticaria in which oedema occurs in the deeper layers of the skin, often on the face, producing transient swellings. It is commonly associated with urticarial weals on other body sites, however angio-oedema without weals may be associated with drug allergy (e.g. ACE inhibitors, NSAIDs) or with C1 esterase inhibitor deficiency (hereditary or acquired). The alarming and disfiguring effects of facial or oropharyngeal angio-oedema usually provoke an acute presentation.

CLINICAL FEATURES

Angio-oedema is usually confined to one area, most commonly lips (**69**), eyelids (**70**), or genitalia. The swellings may be symmetrical or unilateral (**71**) and persist for a few hours to 2–3 days. Affected skin is not red, and itching is usually absent. The tongue and pharynx may be involved. In hereditary angio-oedema there are recurrent swellings of the skin and mucous membranes often associated with vomiting, colicky abdominal pain, and pharyngeal involvement. Angio-oedema may occur as a part of an anaphylaxis reaction.

DIFFERENTIAL DIAGNOSIS

- Erysipelas/cellulitis (p. 126, zone of painful, spreading erythema with fever).
- Lymphoedema (nonpitting oedema with textural changes to the skin).

COMPLICATIONS

- Nausea and vomiting.
- Diarrhoea.
- Anaphylaxis (bronchospasm, laryngeal oedema, hypotension, cardiac dysrhythmia).

INVESTIGATIONS

- The diagnosis is usually made clinically.
- Complement C3, C4 (C4 is lowered in hereditary and acquired C1 esterase inhibitor deficiency). If C4 is low, confirm C1 esterase inhibitor deficiency by specific quantitative and functional assays. C1q is also reduced in acquired C1 esterase inhibitor deficiency.

IMMEDIATE MANAGEMENT

- Stop any precipitating agent (e.g. ACE inhibitor).

Systemic therapy

- In angio-oedema without systemic involvement, treat as urticaria with H1 antihistamines (e.g. cetirizine 10 mg once daily or levocetirizine 5 mg once daily). Sometimes antihistamines need to be given in supranormal doses.
- To terminate an acute attack of hereditary angio-oedema administer C1 esterase inhibitor concentrate or fresh frozen plasma.

Supportive therapy

Treat anaphylaxis with:
- IM or SC epinephrine (adrenaline) 0.5–1.0 mg.
- Slow IV injection of chlorpheniramine 10–20 mg.
- IV hydrocortisone sodium succinate 100–300 mg.
- Oxygen.

LONG-TERM MANAGEMENT ISSUES

In chronic angio-oedema patients develop intermittent episodes of swelling over a prolonged period. Such patients will need to receive maintenance antihistamine therapy and should be under the care of a dermatologist. In hereditary angio-oedema stanozolol, danazol, and tranexamic acid can be used to prevent relapse. Patients with hereditary angio-oedema or a history of anaphylaxis should be encouraged to wear an appropriately marked medical alert amulet. Patients at risk of anaphylaxis should also carry an epinephrine 300 µg autoinjector (e.g. Epipen) and be able to use it appropriately.

69 Angio-oedema. Involvement of the mouth is common and produces swollen lips. This patient also experienced swelling of her tongue but no involvement of the laryngo-pharynx.

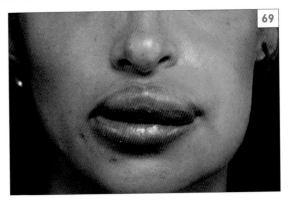

70 Angio-oedema. There is a disfiguring swelling occurring around the eyes due to oedema in the eyelids and surrounding skin.

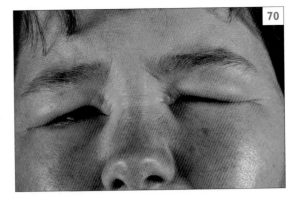

71 Angio-oedema. Angio-oedema can be unilateral.

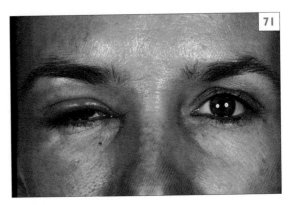

The physical urticarias

In the physical urticarias weals develop following exposure to an environmental trigger. A range of physical stimuli can provoke urticaria including pressure, heat, cold, and UV irradiation. Weals develop within minutes of provocation and resolve after 1–2 hr. The exception to this is delayed pressure urticaria in which lesions take longer to develop and fade. If the stimulus is sufficiently great, or the patient is particularly sensitive, angio-oedema and/or systemic features may occur.

Cold urticaria can be associated with a range of systemic disorders, including EBV and hepatitis infection, lymphoma, cryoglobulinaemia, connective tissue disorders.

CLINICAL FEATURES

The following describes specific physical urticarias:

- Cholinergic urticaria: small, papular weals on the torso are triggered by sweating, usually within minutes of exertion (**72**).
- Symptomatic dermographism: linear weals appear at the site of scratching or rubbing of the skin, e.g. at sites of clothing friction. Itching is often disproportionate to the degree of wealing.
- Cold urticaria: wealing occurs following exposure of the skin to low temperatures, often cold wind and rain.
- Aquagenic urticaria: contact with water of any temperature induces an eruption of multiple small weals.
- Solar urticaria: occurs in the spring and summer and is characterized by confluent urticarial lesions on noncovered skin exposed to strong sunlight (**73**).
- Delayed pressure urticaria: itchy, burning or painful swellings occur 4–6 hr after prolonged pressure to susceptible sites: hands (heavy bag), feet (prolonged standing), buttocks (hard seat), waist (tight clothing) (**74**). Lesions last 8–72 hr.

DIFFERENTIAL DIAGNOSIS

Differential diagnoses will vary according to the type of physical urticaria, e.g.:

Cholinergic urticaria

- Miliaria (p. 204, persistent papules produced as a response to heat).

Symptomatic dermographism

- Pruritus of systemic disease (generalized itch caused by a variety of systemic disorders).

Aquagenic urticaria

- Aquagenic pruritus (itching without urticaria following contact with water).

Solar urticaria

- Polymorphic light eruption (p. 208, itchy papules on uncovered sites developing hours after sun exposure).

COMPLICATIONS

- Headache, palpitations, and syncope (with severe involvement).
- Anaphylaxis (bronchospasm, laryngeal oedema, hypotension, cardiac dysrhythmia).

INVESTIGATIONS

- The diagnosis is usually made clinically.
- Skin contact challenge test, e.g. ice cube for cold urticaria, solar simulator for solar urticaria.

For cold urticaria:

- Blood count, basic chemistry, liver function tests.
- ESR, autoantibodies, cryoglobulins.
- Immunoglobulins and protein electrophoresis.
- Hepatitis B, hepatitis C, and EBV serology.
- Chest radiography.

IMMEDIATE MANAGEMENT

Remove patient from precipitating physical agent.

Topical therapy

- Apply a cooling emollient frequently (e.g. 1% menthol in aqueous cream).

Systemic therapy

- An H1 antihistamine is usually effective (e.g. cetirizine 10 mg once daily or levocetirizine 5 mg once daily). Sometimes antihistamines need to be given in supranormal doses.
- A sedating antihistamine at bedtime is also helpful (e.g. hydroxyzine 25 or 50 mg).

Supportive therapy
Treat anaphylaxis with:
- IM or SC epinephrine (adrenaline) 0.5–1.0 mg.
- Slow IV injection of chlorpheniramine 10–20 mg.
- IV hydrocortisone sodium succinate 100–300 mg.
- Oxygen.

LONG-TERM MANAGEMENT ISSUES
The physical urticarias often persist for months or years and therefore need to be treated as a form of chronic urticaria under the care of a dermatologist. Induction of tolerance in some cases can be achieved by repeated, graduated exposure to the precipitating factor. Systemic immunosuppressants can be used in cases of severe physical urticaria. Patients who develop significant systemic symptoms following episodes of physical urticaria should be encouraged to wear an appropriately marked medical alert amulet.

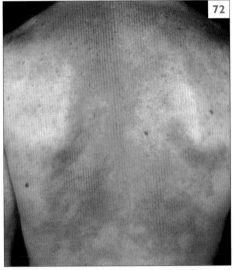

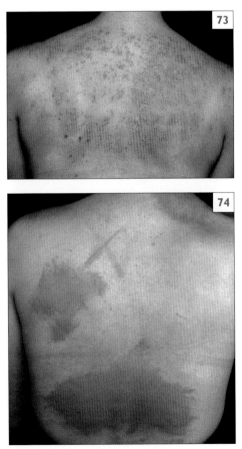

72 Cholinergic urticaria. Weals and urticated erythema involving the back and chest develop shortly after exercise.

73 Solar urticaria. Erythema with weals developed on the exposed skin of this woman's back following several minutes exposure to strong sunlight. Note the clearly delineated margins of her dress.

74 Delayed pressure urticaria. Weals appear at the site of pressure on the skin. This patient also displays positive dermographism, in which linear weals develop at sites of skin scratching.

Urticarial vasculitis

Urticarial vasculitis is a type III hypersensitivity vasculitis in which urticarial weals develop rather than palpable purpura. The eruption often develops acutely and is sometimes associated with systemic symptoms.

CLINICAL FEATURES

The weals of urticarial vasculitis typically last longer than in ordinary urticaria (greater than 24 hr) and may resolve to leave bruising or hyperpigmentation. The lesions are often generalized and may burn or be painful as well as itchy (**75, 76**). Angio-oedema is present in approximately 40% of cases. Urticarial vasculitis has been associated with hepatitis infection, systemic lupus erythematosus (SLE), Sjögren's syndrome, haematological malignancies, chronic obstructive pulmonary disease, and some drugs (e.g. diltiazem).

DIFFERENTIAL DIAGNOSIS

- Acute urticaria (p. 56, itchy weals which last for less than 24 hr).
- Erythema multiforme (p. 144, urticated or blistered target-like lesions especially on acral skin).
- Bullous pemphigoid, pre-bullous phase (p. 66, itchy, urticated plaques).

COMPLICATIONS

- Arthralgia and arthritis.
- Abdominal pain, nausea, vomiting.
- Fever.
- Renal impairment.

INVESTIGATIONS
Vasculitis screen

- Blood count, basic chemistry, liver function tests (useful as indicators of general health and important as a baseline for the monitoring of systemic therapy).
- ESR, CRP (elevated).
- Urinalysis (haematuria indicates renal involvement).
- Antinuclear antibody (ANA), anti-dsDNA, -Sm, -ribonuclear protein (-RNP), -Ro(SS-A), -La(SS-B) antibodies (to exclude LE).
- Rheumatoid factor, antineutrophil cytoplasmic antibody (ANCA).

- Complement C3, C4 (low C3, C4, and C1q occur in hypocomplementaemic urticarial vasculitis, which carries a worse prognosis).
- Immunoglobulins, serum protein electrophoresis, cryoglobulins.
- Throat swab, antistreptolysin O titre (ASOT), blood cultures, hepatitis B and hepatitis C serology, HIV serology (if indicated).
- Skin biopsy for histopathology (leucocytoclastic vasculitis, prominent upper dermal oedema).
- Skin biopsy for direct immunofluorescence (vascular deposition of immunoglobulin).

IMMEDIATE MANAGEMENT

Exclude the presence of systemic vasculitis.

Systemic therapy

- Supranormal doses of H1 antihistamines may be effective in settling the eruption (e.g. levocetirizine 5 mg twice daily).
- Many cases will require a short course of oral corticosteroids in order to gain symptomatic control (e.g. prednisolone 20–30 mg/day for 1–2 weeks).

LONG-TERM MANAGEMENT ISSUES

Urticarial vasculitis tends to run a relatively protracted course (1–3 years) and patients need long-term follow-up by a dermatologist. Many patients require maintenance treatment with an immunosuppressant drug (e.g. azathioprine, mycophenolate mofetil) plus intermittent courses of oral corticosteroids. Other second-line drugs which can be useful in urticarial vasculitis are methotrexate, colchicine, dapsone, and antimalarials.

75 Urticarial vasculitis. These persistent weals in a patient with SLE showed the features of vasculitis on skin biopsy. The patient described burning, rather than itching.

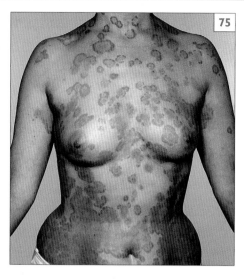

76 Urticarial vasculitis. The legs of the same patient in **75**. The weals in urticarial vasculitis resemble those in ordinary urticaria, but they persist for more than 24 hr and resolve with bruising.

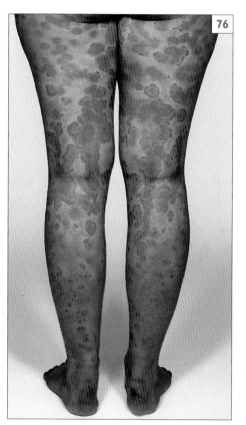

Blistering diseases

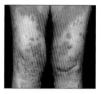
Bullous pemphigoid

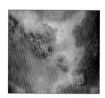
Epidermolysis bullosa acquisita

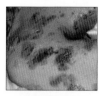
Pemphigus vulgaris and pemphigus foliaceous

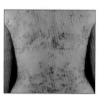
Linear IgA bullous dermatosis

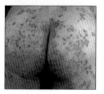
Dermatitis herpetiformis

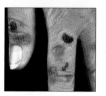
Porphyria cutanea tarda

Bullous pemphigoid

Bullous pemphigoid (BP) is a subepidermal, autoimmune blistering skin disease which occurs predominantly in middle-aged or elderly individuals. Blistering is caused by antibodies directed against proteins involved in adhesion of epidermis to underlying dermis (BP antigen 180 and BP antigen 230). Severe itching or the development of blisters usually precipitates an acute presentation.

CLINICAL FEATURES

Prior to the appearance of blisters there is often a prodrome of itchy, urticated erythema which can be figurate in appearance (**77**). This may persist for several weeks before tense blisters of varying size arise on inflamed skin (**78, 79**). The main areas of involvement are the arms, legs, flexures, and lower abdomen. Nikolsky's sign is negative. Rupture of blisters produces large amounts of serous exudate. Loss of the blister roof will expose the dermis which can become secondarily infected. Mucosal involvement is unusual in ordinary BP, however mucous membrane pemphigoid (MMP) is characterized by blisters, erosions, and scarring on ocular, buccal, and genital mucosae.

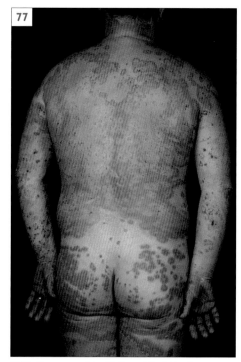

77 Bullous pemphigoid. Pemphigoid in the pre-bullous phase with multiple, annular plaques on the torso and limbs. Lesional skin is red, urticated, and itchy. There are a few blisters on the arms.

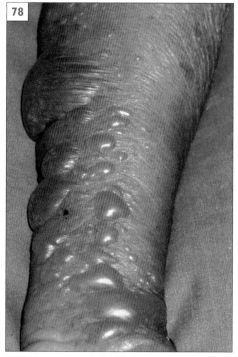

78 Bullous pemphigoid. The blisters are large, tense, and develop on red, inflamed skin.

DIFFERENTIAL DIAGNOSIS

- Bullous impetigo (p. 118, erythema, tense blisters, and honey-coloured crust).
- Oedema blisters (p. 96, rapid accumulation of oedema at dependent sites producing blisters).
- Bullous erythema multiforme (p. 144, urticated or blistered target-like lesions especially on acral skin).
- Stevens–Johnson syndrome/toxic epidermal necrolysis (p. 230, widespread blistering with mucous membrane involvement).
- Linear IgA bullous dermatosis (p. 76, itchy erythema with large tense blisters).
- Epidermolysis bullosa acquisita (p. 74, blisters occurring at sites of mechanical trauma).
- Dermatitis herpetiformis (p. 72, itchy vesicles on extensor surfaces).
- Pemphigus vulgaris (p. 70, vesicles, bullae, and erosions, usually involves the mouth).
- Pemphigoid gestationis (p. 214, itchy erythema and blisters in second or third trimester of pregnancy).
- Bullous lupus erythematosus (p. 108, blisters in acute lupus erythematosus).

COMPLICATIONS

- Secondary bacterial infection (may lead to systemic sepsis).
- Fluid and protein loss (with widespread blistering).
- Anaemia (with widespread blistering).

In MMP:
- Malnutrition (impaired ability to eat and drink with severe oral involvement).
- Corneal scarring (with ocular involvement).
- Dysuria, dyspareunia, and genital scarring (with genital involvement).

INVESTIGATIONS

- Blood count, basic chemistry, liver function tests (indicators of general health; baseline for monitoring systemic therapy).
- Skin biopsy across a blister margin for histopathology (subepidermal blister with an eosinophil-rich inflammatory cell infiltrate in the dermis and blister).
- Skin biopsy of perilesional skin for direct immunofluorescence (linear deposition of C3 and IgG along the dermoepidermal junction).
- Serum for indirect immunofluorescence (antibody binds to the roof of salt-split skin).
- Skin swab for bacteriology (if secondary infection is suspected).

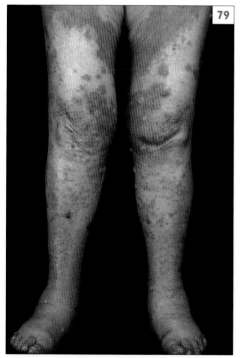

79 Bullous pemphigoid. Extensive BP with numerous blisters within large areas of erythema.

IMMEDIATE MANAGEMENT
Topical therapy
- Tense blisters should be decompressed by sterile aspiration.
- Potassium permanganate soaks once daily to denuded areas.
- Nonadherent dressings to denuded areas.
- General emollient therapy.
- Corticosteroid ointment, twice per day (use for restricted period):
    trunk and limbs: potent or
    superpotent.

Systemic therapy
- Adequate analgesia.
- Systemic corticosteroids are usually necessary, e.g. prednisolone 0.5–1 mg/kg/day, reducing with response.
- Oral antibiotics for secondary bacterial infection.

Supportive therapy
Patients with BP may need to be admitted to hospital for the following:
- Bed rest and intensive topical therapy (see above).
- Initiation of systemic therapy.
- Monitoring of vital signs (pulse rate, blood pressure, temperature).
- Monitoring of fluid balance.
- Administration of intravenous fluids, if required.
- Analgesia.

LONG-TERM MANAGEMENT ISSUES
Prednisolone should be tapered with response and a steroid-sparing agent introduced, such as azathioprine 1–3 mg/kg/day in divided doses or mycophenolate mofetil 500–1500 mg twice per day. Minocycline 100 mg once daily has been used to control mild BP. Prolonged use of systemic corticosteroids requires on-going screening for diabetes, hypertension, and osteoporosis. Osteoporosis prophylaxis is recommended. Gastric protection with a proton pump inhibitor is often needed (e.g. omeprazole 20 mg once daily). Patients with BP need to be under regular follow-up by a dermatologist.

Pemphigus vulgaris and pemphigus foliaceous

Pemphigus is an intraepithelial, autoimmune blistering disease mediated by circulating autoantibodies which disrupt keratinocyte adhesion. In pemphigus vulgaris the target intercellular adhesion molecule is desmoglein 3, which is found predominantly in the lower parts of the epidermis. In pemphigus foliaceous the target is desmoglein 1 in the upper parts of the epidermis. Involvement of the oral mucous membranes in PV can cause considerable local morbidity and problems with nutrition, while extensive skin involvement may lead to serious systemic complications, such as sepsis.

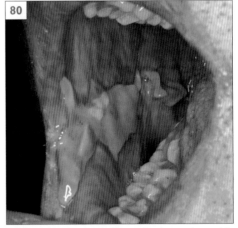

80 Pemphigus vulgaris. There is a large ulcer with slough on the buccal mucosa. PV often starts in the mouth.

CLINICAL FEATURES

PV usually presents with oral blisters and erosions (**80**). These are often irregularly shaped and situated on the buccal or palatal surfaces. Oral involvement may be the sole manifestation of PV or predate, by several months, the appearance of lesions on skin and other mucosal sites. Cutaneous involvement (**81–83**) is characterized by flaccid blisters and painful erosions which may be localized or generalized, especially affecting the scalp, face, axillae, groin, and pressure points. Nikolsky's sign is positive. PF rarely involves mucosae but generally presents with small, flaccid bullae on the face, scalp, neck, and torso (**84**).

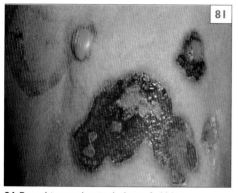

81 Pemphigus vulgaris. A deroofed blister showing exposed underlying dermis. The intact blister above is secondarily infected and contains pus.

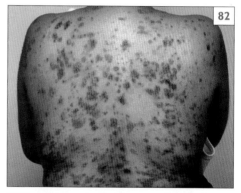

82 Pemphigus vulgaris. Numerous inflamed lesions on the back, some of which have become eroded. No obvious intact blisters are seen, which is typical for PV.

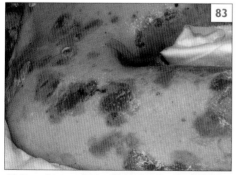

83 Pemphigus vulgaris. This patient, severely ill with PV, has multiple eroded areas on the torso and limbs. The patient was admitted to hospital and required supportive treatment as well as intensive immunosuppressant therapy.

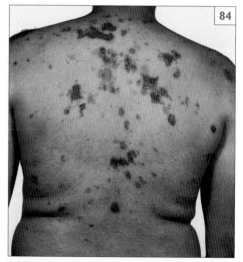

84 Pemphigus foliaceous. There are numerous discrete blisters and erosions on the back occurring in a 'seborrhoeic' distribution.

However the blisters rupture easily in PF and give way to erosions and areas of scaling and crusting (**85, 86**). Paraneoplastic pemphigus presents as a polymorphic eruption of lichenoid rash, target-like lesions, blisters, and mucosal involvement.

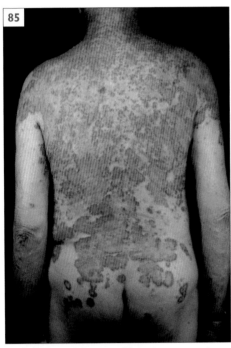

85 Pemphigus foliaceous. There is an extensive eruption of annular lesions. No blisters or erosions are seen.

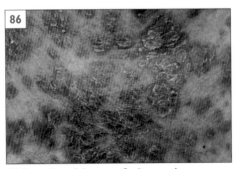

86 Pemphigus foliaceous. Scaling can be prominent in PF.

DIFFERENTIAL DIAGNOSIS
Pemphigus vulgaris
- Bullous erythema multiforme (p. 144, orogenital ulceration associated with urticated or blistered target-like lesions especially on acral skin).
- PF (see above).
- Mucous membrane pemphigoid (p. 66, erosions and scarring of mucosae, blisters on skin).
- Stevens–Johnson syndrome/toxic epidermal necrolysis (p. 230, widespread blistering with mucous membrane involvement).

Pemphigus foliaceous
- PV (see above).
- Impetigo (p. 118, areas of erythema with overlying honey-coloured crust).
- Seborrhoeic dermatitis (p. 20, erythema and scaling of the face, scalp, and chest).
- Subacute cutaneous lupus erythematosus (p. 110, annular and polycyclic eruption on upper torso).

Oral pemphigus
- Recurrent aphthous stomatitis (recurrent large mouth ulcers).
- Behçet's disease (orogenital ulceration and uveitis).
- Mucous membrane pemphigoid (p. 66, erosions and scarring of mucosae, blisters on skin).
- Erosive oral lichen planus (p. 36, mouth ulcers with white reticulate changes on buccal mucosae).
- Angina bullosa haemorrhagica (bullous purpura on oral mucosae).

COMPLICATIONS
- Secondary bacterial infection (may lead to systemic sepsis).
- Excessive fluid, heat, and protein loss (with widespread blistering).
- Malnutrition (impaired ability to eat and drink with severe oral involvement).
- Anaemia (with widespread blistering).
- Corneal scarring (with ocular involvement).
- Dysuria, dyspareunia, and genital scarring (with genital involvement).

INVESTIGATIONS

- Blood count, basic chemistry, liver function tests (indicators of general health; baseline for monitoring systemic therapy).
- Skin biopsy across a blister margin for histopathology (PV – lower epidermal acantholysis with intraepidermal blistering; PF – upper epidermal acantholysis with subcorneal clefting).
- Skin biopsy of perilesional skin for direct immunofluorescence (IgG deposited on the surface of the keratinocytes in both PV and PF).
- Serum for indirect immunofluorescence (antibody binds to the surface of keratinocytes in both PV and PF: antibody titre in PV reflects disease activity).
- Skin swab for bacteriology (if secondary infection is suspected).
- ELISA for antibodies to desmogleins 1 and 3.

IMMEDIATE MANAGEMENT
Topical therapy

- Oral involvement: steroid mouthwashes.
- General emollient therapy.
- Corticosteroid ointment, twice per day (use for restricted period):
    trunk and limbs: potent or superpotent.
- Potassium permanganate soaks once daily to eroded areas.
- Nonadherent dressings to denuded areas.

Systemic therapy
- Adequate analgesia.
- Systemic corticosteroids are usually necessary, e.g. prednisolone 0.5–1 mg/kg/day, reducing with response.
- Oral antibiotics for secondary infection.

Supportive therapy
Patients with severe pemphigus may need to be admitted to hospital for the following:
- Bed rest and intensive topical therapy (see above).
- Initiation of systemic therapy.
- Monitoring of vital signs (pulse rate, blood pressure, temperature).
- Monitoring of fluid balance.
- Administration of intravenous fluids, if required.
- Supportive nutrition, including nasogastric feeding.
- Monitoring of body temperature regulation.
- Analgesia.
- IV therapy (see below).

LONG-TERM MANAGEMENT ISSUES
PV is more aggressive than PF and tends to require greater immunosuppressive therapy. Generalized PV which is not responding to oral corticosteroid may be controlled by intravenous pulses of methylprednisolone 500 mg or 1 g given over 3 hr for 3 consecutive days and repeated every 21–30 days until remission has been achieved. Adjuvant immunosuppressant therapy is often also needed, e.g. azathioprine 1–3 mg/kg/day or mycophenolate mofetil 500–1500 mg twice per day. Alternatively, cyclophosphamide can be used in combination with pulsed methyl-prednisolone, e.g. IV cyclophosphamide 500 mg given once every 21–30 days with 50 mg oral cyclophosphamide daily until remission has been achieved. In recalcitrant pemphigus, intravenous immunoglobulin can be effective: 0.4 g/kg/day for 5 consecutive days, repeated monthly for 3 consecutive months. PF can usually be controlled with lower requirements of corticosteroid and immunosuppressants, compared to PV. Dapsone 100–300 mg once daily can also be effective in PF. In unrespon-sive pemphigus, remission can be achieved with rituximab, a chimeric anti-CD20 monoclonal antibody. Prolonged use of systemic corti-costeroids requires on-going screening for diabetes, hypertension, and osteoporosis. Osteoporosis prophylaxis is recommended. Gastric protection with a proton pump inhibitor is often needed (e.g. omeprazole 20 mg once daily). Patients with pemphigus must be under the care of a dermatologist, but other specialists, such as oral physicians and ophthalmologists, may also need to be consulted.

Dermatitis herpetiformis

Dermatitis herpetiformis (DH) is an auto-immune blistering skin disease which is associated with a gluten-sensitive enteropathy. Typically, DH develops in the second to fourth decades. The enteropathy usually presents with diarrhoea, bloating, abdominal pain, and can lead to malabsorption. Very rarely it is associated with small bowel lymphoma. Although DH tends to follow a chronic course, the intense itching which accompanies the eruption often causes the patient to seek an urgent opinion.

CLINICAL FEATURES
Groups of red papules and vesicles develop symmetrically on the extensor surfaces, especially buttocks, knees, and elbows (**87, 88**). Since DH is so itchy the vesicles are often ruptured by scratching (**89**). Other sites of involvement include the scapular and sacral areas, hairline, and scalp. The mucous membranes are not usually involved. Occasionally the lesions may be urticarial or bullous.

DIFFERENTIAL DIAGNOSIS
- Atopic dermatitis (p. 8, eczema as part of the atopic diathesis).
- Prurigo (excoriated and lichenified papules from chronic pruritus).
- Scabies (p. 162, widespread itching with burrows which can occasionally blister).
- Erythema multiforme (p. 144, urticated or blistered target-like lesions especially on acral skin).
- Epidermolysis bullosa acquisita (p. 74, blisters occurring at sites of mechanical trauma).
- Bullous pemphigoid (p. 66, itchy erythema with large tense blisters).

COMPLICATIONS
- Secondary bacterial infection.

INVESTIGATIONS
- Blood count, basic chemistry, liver function tests (indicators of general health; baseline for monitoring systemic therapy).
- Glucose-6-phosphate dehydrogenase (G-6-PD) (must be tested prior to starting dapsone).
- Anti-transglutaminase antibodies (positive in gluten sensitivity).
- Skin biopsy across a blister margin for histopathology (clefting at the dermoepidermal junction with microabscesses in the dermal papillae composed of neutrophils and eosinophils).
- Skin biopsy of uninvolved skin for direct immunofluorescence (granular deposit of IgA in the dermal papillae and a linear deposit of IgA along the dermoepidermal junction).
- Skin swab for bacteriology (if secondary infection is suspected).

IMMEDIATE MANAGEMENT
Systemic therapy
- If the G-6-PD levels are normal give dapsone at a starting dose of 1–2 mg/kg/day (100–150 mg). Thereafter maintain dapsone at a dose of 50–200 mg once daily according to response. G-6-PD deficiency results in severe dapsone-induced haemolysis.

LONG-TERM MANAGEMENT ISSUES
Following the introduction of dapsone improvement is often dramatic with clearance of lesions and the itch within a few days. A small bowel biopsy is needed to investigate the presence of a gluten-sensitive enteropathy. All patients should be commenced on a gluten-free diet which will improve the gastrointestinal pathology (dapsone is ineffective in controlling enteropathy) and, in some cases, may control the skin features. Wheat, barley, and rye contain gluten and should be avoided; oats, rice, and maize are gluten-free and can therefore be eaten. Methaemoglobinaemia can arise due to low G-6-PD levels in patients treated with dapsone, therefore regular monitoring of the blood count and methaemoglobin is necessary. Haemolysis is also a common complication of dapsone therapy. If dapsone is not tolerated then sulfapyridine, at 500–2000 mg/day, can be used instead. Sulfamethoxypyridazine 250–1500 mg/day is an alternative, if the patient is intolerant of sulfapyridine. DH patients will need to be under the care of a dermatologist and a gastroenterologist.

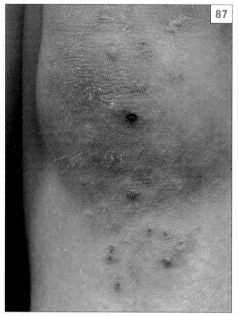

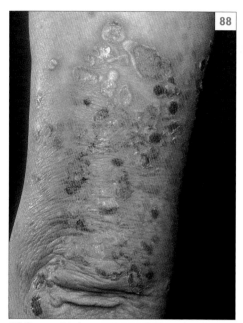

87 Dermatitis herpetiformis. A cluster of papules and vesicles over the knee, a typical site for DH.

88 Dermatitis herpetiformis. DH on the elbow with erythema, excoriated blisters, erosions, and evidence of secondary bacterial infection.

89 Dermatitis herpetiformis. Extensive DH on the buttocks. Scratching has eliminated the vesicles.

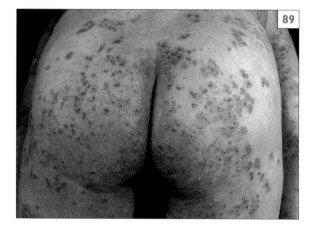

Epidermolysis bullosa acquisita

Epidermolysis bullosa acquisita (EBA) is a rare, acquired, autoimmune condition in which blisters are induced at sites of mechanical trauma. It can occur at any age. Cases have been associated with Crohn's disease, ulcerative colitis, and systemic lupus erthematosus. In most patients there are antibodies directed against type VII collagen, the major component of anchoring fibrils which bind epidermis to dermis.

CLINICAL FEATURES

Tense, haemorrhagic blisters and erosions develop at sites of skin trauma (**90, 91**): fingers and backs of the hands, elbows, buttocks, sacrum and tops of the feet. The blisters heal with hyperpigmentation, scarring, and milia (**92**). In some cases the mechanobullous picture is less clear and the condition resembles bullous pemphigoid with blisters in the flexures, on the proximal limbs and torso (**90**). Involvement of the nails leads to dystrophy. Erosions and blisters may develop in the mouth, larynx, and oesophagus.

DIFFERENTIAL DIAGNOSIS

- Bullous pemphigoid (p. 66, itchy erythema with large tense blisters).
- Mucous membrane pemphigoid (p. 66, erosions and scarring of mucosae, blisters on skin).
- Porphyria cutanea tarda (p. 78, skin fragility and blisters on exposed sites).
- Erythema multiforme (p. 144, urticated or blistered target-like lesions especially on acral skin).
- Dermatitis herpetiformis (p. 72, itchy vesicles on extensor surfaces).

COMPLICATIONS

- Secondary bacterial infection (may lead to systemic sepsis).
- Excessive fluid, heat, and protein loss (with widespread blistering).
- Malnutrition (impaired ability to eat and drink with oro-oesophageal involvement).
- Laryngeal stenosis.
- Oesophageal stricture.
- Anaemia (with widespread blistering).

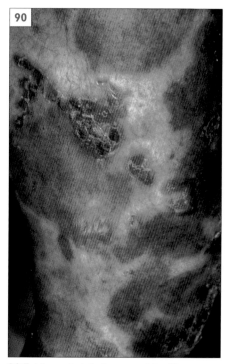

90 Epidermolysis bullosa acquisita. There are blisters and erosions on large areas of urticated erythema, resembling BP.

- Corneal scarring (with ocular involvement).
- Dysuria, dyspareunia, and genital scarring (with genital involvement).

INVESTIGATIONS

- Blood count, basic chemistry, liver function tests (indicators of general health; baseline for monitoring systemic therapy).
- Skin biopsy across a blister margin for histopathology (subepidermal blister: noninflammatory in some cases, associated with a neutrophil-rich infiltrate in other cases).
- Skin biopsy of perilesional skin for direct immunofluorescence (a linear deposit of IgG and C3 at the basement membrane zone).
- Serum for indirect immunofluorescence (antibody will bind to the floor of salt-split skin in approximately 50% of patients).
- Skin swab for bacteriology (if secondary infection is suspected).

91 Epidermolysis bullosa acquisita. There are patches of erythema over the knees containing erosions and milia. It is typical for epidermolysis bullosa acquisita to be limited to sites of trauma.

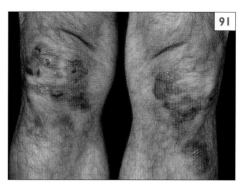

92 Epidermolysis bullosa acquisita. The knuckles are another common site of involvement. In this patient there are multiple milia on a background of redness.

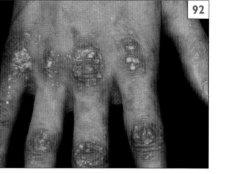

IMMEDIATE MANAGEMENT

Topical therapy

- The blisters should be decompressed by sterile aspiration.
- General emollient therapy.
- Potassium permanganate soaks once daily to denuded areas.
- Nonadherent dressings to denuded areas.
- Corticosteroid ointment, twice per day (use for a restricted period):
  trunk and limbs: potent or superpotent. (helpful if there is an inflammatory component).

Systemic therapy

- Oral corticosteroids are sometimes helpful, e.g. prednisolone 0.5–1 mg/kg once daily, reducing with response.
- Oral antibiotics for secondary bacterial infection.

LONG-TERM MANAGEMENT ISSUES

EBA is often difficult to treat successfully. An immunosuppressive regime is generally used with a combination of corticosteroids and a steroid-sparing agent, such as azathioprine, ciclosporin or mycophenolate mofetil. Intravenous immunoglobulin can also be helpful. Prolonged use of systemic corticosteroids requires screening for diabetes, hypertension, and osteoporosis. Osteoporosis prophylaxis is recommended. Gastric protection with a proton pump inhibitor is often needed (e.g. omeprazole 20 mg once daily). In recalcitrant EBA, remission can be achieved with rituximab, a chimeric anti-CD20 monoclonal antibody. Patients with EBA must be under the care of a dermatologist, but other specialists, such as oral physicians, gastroenterologists, and ophthalmologists, may also need to be consulted.

Linear IgA bullous dermatosis

Linear IgA bullous dermatosis (LABD) is a rare, autoimmune bullous disease which presents with subepidermal blisters, in the same way as bullous pemphigoid. Drug-induced LABD has been reported with a number of agents, including vancomycin, diclofenac, and other NSAIDs. There is also an association with Crohn's disease, ulcerative colitis, and malignancy (especially lymphoid, but also solid organ tumours).

CLINICAL FEATURES

The eruption presents suddenly with urticated plaques which develop into vesicles and blisters (**93, 94**). The characteristic lesions of LABD are annular with blisters and vesicles arranged along the margins to form rosettes. Itching and a burning pain are common. The disease is often widespread with involvement of the torso, limbs, face, and scalp. Mucosal surfaces are commonly affected with mouth ulcers, nasal crusting, and sore eyes.

DIFFERENTIAL DIAGNOSIS

- Bullous pemphigoid (p. 66, itchy erythema with large tense blisters).
- Pemphigus vulgaris (p. 68, vesicles, bullae, and erosions, usually involves the mouth).
- Erythema multiforme (p. 144, urticated or blistered target-like lesions especially on acral skin).
- Bullous lupus erythematosus (p. 108, blisters in acute lupus erythematosus).
- Epidermolysis bullosa acquisita (p. 74, blisters occurring at sites of mechanical trauma).
- Dermatitis herpetiformis (p. 72, itchy vesicles on extensor surfaces).

COMPLICATIONS

- Secondary bacterial infection (may lead to systemic sepsis).
- Excessive fluid, heat, and protein loss (with widespread blistering).
- Malnutrition (impaired ability to eat and drink with severe oral involvement).
- Anaemia (with widespread blistering).
- Ocular scarring.

INVESTIGATIONS

- Blood count, basic chemistry, liver function tests (useful as indicators of general health and important as a baseline for the monitoring of systemic therapy).
- G-6-PD (G-6-PD deficiency results in severe dapsone-induced haemolysis).
- Skin biopsy across a blister margin for histopathology (subepidermal blistering with an eosinophil-rich infiltrate; in some blisters, neutrophils predominate and dermal microabscesses are seen).
- Skin biopsy of perilesional skin for direct immunofluorescence (linear deposition of IgA along the dermoepidermal junction).
- Serum for indirect immunofluorescence (IgA basement membrane zone autoantibodies are positive in approximately 30% of adult cases; on salt-split skin antibodies bind to epidermal side).
- Skin swab for bacteriology (if secondary infection is suspected).

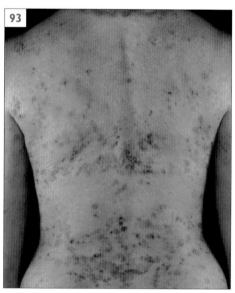

93 Linear IgA bullous dermatosis. Multiple urticated, excoriated papules. At this time, no intact blisters were present.

IMMEDIATE MANAGEMENT
Topical therapy
- The blisters should be decompressed by sterile aspiration.
- General emollient therapy.
- Nonadherent dressings to denuded areas.
- Corticosteroid ointment, twice per day (use for restricted period):
    trunk and limbs: potent or superpotent.

Systemic therapy
- If the G-6-PD levels are normal give dapsone at a starting dose of 1–2 mg/kg/day (100–150 mg). Thereafter maintain dapsone at a dose of 50–200 mg once daily according to response.

LONG-TERM MANAGEMENT ISSUES
Methaemoglobinaemia can arise due to low G-6-PD levels in patients treated with dapsone, therefore regular monitoring of the blood count and methaemoglobin is necessary. Haemolysis is also a common complication of dapsone therapy. If dapsone is not tolerated then sulfapyridine, at 500–2000 mg/day can be used instead. Sulfamethoxypyridazine 250–1500 mg/day is an alternative, if the patient is intolerant of sulfapyridine. As with other autoimmune bullous dermatoses, patients with LABD need to be under regular follow-up by a dermatologist. LABD often remits spontaneously after 3–6 years.

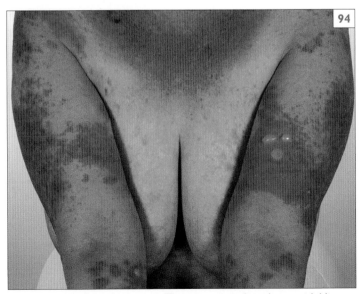

94 Linear IgA bullous dermatosis. There is urticated erythema with blisters on the upper arms.

Porphyria cutanea tarda

Porphyria cutanea tarda (PCT) is the commonest of the porphyrias. It is caused by decreased activity of the hepatic enzyme uroporphyrinogen decarboxylase leading to an accumulation of porphyrins. Circulating porphyrins are activated by visible light resulting in a phototoxic reaction which causes fragility of exposed skin. PCT is usually acquired (sporadic form) and is often associated with liver disease. There is also an association with haemochromatosis, hepatitis B and C infection, and HIV infection. The clinical manifestations of PCT can be precipitated by excess alcohol intake or the ingestion of therapeutic oestrogens. Although the skin features can develop suddenly, PCT is not associated with acute systemic symptoms, such as those seen in variegate porphyria.

CLINICAL FEATURES
Blisters and erosions occur on the sun-exposed skin of the hands and forearms and on the face (**95**). Blisters heal with crusting to leave atrophic scars and milia. Patients also notice increased skin fragility of the hands and forearms (**96**). Although patients with PCT are abnormally photosensitive they rarely associate the development of lesions with sun exposure. Involved skin is often hyperpigmented and sometimes shows hypertrichosis.

DIFFERENTIAL DIAGNOSIS
- Drug-induced pseudoporphyria (sun-induced skin fragility produced by drugs, e.g. furosemide).
- Variegate porphyria (an acute porphyria with same skin features as PCT).
- Bullous pemphigoid (p. 66, itchy erythema with large tense blisters).
- Epidermolysis bullosa acquisita (p. 74, blisters occurring at sites of mechanical trauma).
- Bullous lupus erythematosus (p. 108, blisters in acute lupus erythematosus).

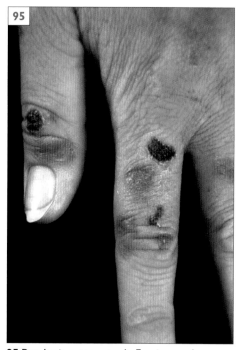

95 Porphyria cutanea tarda. Erosions and scars on the dorsal aspect of the fingers.

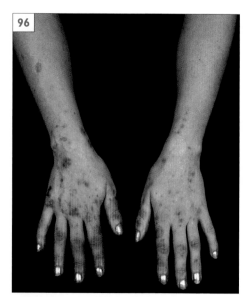

96 Porphyria cutanea tarda. Signs of old blisters and skin fragility on the backs of the hands and wrists, the typical sites of involvement.

COMPLICATIONS

- Secondary bacterial infection.
- Signs of iron overload.
- PCT is NOT associated with the systemic features of an acute porphyria (abdominal pain, fever, neuropathies, confusion, psychosis, coma).

INVESTIGATIONS

- Blood count, basic chemistry, liver function tests (liver transaminases are often elevated).
- International normalized ratio (INR) (raised in liver failure).
- Ferritin (raised; iron overload is common).
- Hepatitis B and C serology.
- HIV test (if indicated).
- Ultrasonography of liver (to exclude chronic liver disease or cirrhosis).
- Porphyrin analysis of plasma, urine, and faeces:
- Urine: increased uroporphyrin.
- Faeces: increased isocoproporphyrin.
- Plasma: spectrofluorimetry peak at 615–620 nm.
- Skin biopsy across a blister margin for histopathology (subepidermal blister with minimal inflammatory infiltrate and festooning of the dermal papillae).
- Skin biopsy across a blister margin for direct immunofluorescence (IgM and IgG along the dermoepidermal junction.

IMMEDIATE MANAGEMENT
Topical therapy

- Photoprotection advice: sunlight avoidance, photoprotective clothing and hat, use of a broad-spectrum, high protection factor topical sunscreen.

Systemic therapy

- Discontinue any precipitating agent (e.g. alcohol, therapeutic oestrogens).
- In order to reduce iron stores therapeutic venesection is the treatment of choice: one unit of blood is removed every 1–2 weeks until the haemoglobin falls to 11–12 g/dl.
- If venesection is not tolerated then treat with oral chloroquine phosphate 125–250 mg twice per week or hydroxychloroquine sulfate 200–400 mg twice per week.

LONG-TERM MANAGEMENT ISSUES

At presentation approximately one-half of patients with PCT will have liver disease and 15% will have cirrhosis. Patients have a significantly increased risk of developing hepatocellular carcinoma. As well as identifying any exogenous factors which may inhibit hepatic uroporphyrinogen decarboxylase it is important to consider subclinical genetic haemochromatosis, and test for the Cys282Tyr haemochromatosis mutation.

Vascular diseases

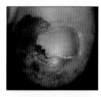 **Small vessel vasculitis**

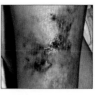 **Calciphylaxis**

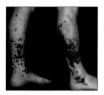 **Polyarteritis nodosa**

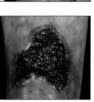 **Pyoderma gangrenosum**

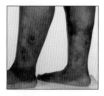 **Cutaneous embolism**

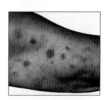 **Sweet's syndrome**

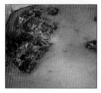 **Widespread cutaneous necrosis**

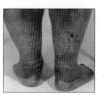 **Dependency syndrome**

Small vessel vasculitis

The term small vessel vasculitis (SVV) can be used to describe a range of disorders all characterized by microvascular inflammation occurring in the skin and, often, in other organs as well. It is also called 'leucocytoclastic vasculitis' (indicating the histopathological changes) and 'hypersensitivity vasculitis' (indicating the allergic nature of some cases). SVV may occur as a purely cutaneous problem, however examination and investigation to exclude systemic involvement is mandatory. Disorders which may be accompanied by cutaneous SVV are: Henoch–Schönlein purpura (plus gastrointestinal, renal, and joint involvement); systemic vasculitides (e.g. microscopic polyangiitis, Churg–Strauss syndrome); systemic infections (e.g. *Meningococcus*, *Streptococcus*, hepatitis B); connective tissue disorders (e.g. systemic lupus erythematosus, Sjögren's syndrome, rheumatoid arthritis); drug allergy; type II and III mixed cryoglobulinaemia (caused by hepatitis C, hepatitis B, HIV infections, rheumatoid arthritis, systemic lupus erythematosus); internal malignancy.

CLINICAL FEATURES

The cardinal sign of SVV is purpura (nonblanching erythema) which is palpable and most usually occurs on the lower legs. The lesions initially develop as tiny dark red petechiae which appear individually or in crops. These evolve into purpuric papules (**97, 98**) which may become vesicular or pustular. Palpable purpura can be sore, painful or itchy. Multiple purpuric lesions can coalesce to form large ecchymoses or haemorrhagic blisters (**99, 100**). Extensive lower leg involvement is associated with regional oedema. In severe cases purpura can occur on other sites, most usually the arms and dependent areas. SVV can also present with urticarial plaques (urticarial vasculitis, see p. 62) and target-like lesions. In Henoch–Schönlein purpura the purpura occurs predominantly over the buttocks and lower limbs. In cryoglobulinaemic vasculitis, distal ischaemia and necrosis may occur in conjunction with palpable purpura.

DIFFERENTIAL DIAGNOSIS

- Capillaritis (red or brown patches containing 'cayenne pepper' spots).
- Thrombocytopenic petechiae (pinpoint macular purpura).
- Cutaneous emboli (p. 86, purpuric lesions on acral skin with livedo reticularis).
- Thrombophilia disorders (large stellate or retiform purpuric patches).

COMPLICATIONS

- Fever and malaise.
- Hypertension.
- Arthritis.
- Haematuria and renal insufficiency.
- Abdominal pain and gastrointestinal bleeding.
- Neuropathy.
- Cerebrovascular insufficiency.

INVESTIGATIONS

Vasculitis screen

- Blood count (eosinophilia is characteristic of Churg–Strauss syndrome; neutrophilia, thrombocytosis, and normocytic anaemia occur in systemic polyarteritis nodosa).
- Basic chemistry, liver function tests (impaired renal function indicates renal vasculitis).
- ESR, CRP (inflammatory markers are raised).
- Urinalysis (haematuria and proteinuria indicate renal vasculitis).
- ANCA (p-ANCA (anti-myeloperoxidase: -MPO) is positive in 60% of microscopic polyangiitis and 40% Churg–Strauss syndrome; c-ANCA (anti-serine proteinase 3: -PR3) is positive in 90% Wegener's granulomatosis and 30% of microscopic polyangiitis).
- ANA, complement, anti-dsDNA, -Sm, -Ro(SS-A), -La(SS-B), -RNP antibodies (to exclude systemic lupus erythematosus).
- Rheumatoid factor (raised in rheumatoid arthritis and mixed essential cryoglobulinaemia).
- Cryoglobulins (raised in cryoglobulinaemia).
- Throat swab, ASOT, blood cultures (HSP can be triggered by an upper respiratory tract infection; SVV can be caused by meningococcal or other bacterial septicaemia).

97 Small vessel vasculitis. There is an eruption of tiny, dark red lesions on the lower legs and feet. Vasculitis in this patient was triggered by streptococcal pharyngitis.

98 Small vessel vasculitis. Same patient as in **97**. SVV consists of palpable purpura.

99 Small vessel vasculitis. This patient developed a vasculitis as part of a hypersensitivity reaction to a drug. The purpura is extensive and confluent.

100 Small vessel vasculitis. Same patient as in **99**. The purpura is blistering, a complication of intense vascular inflammation.

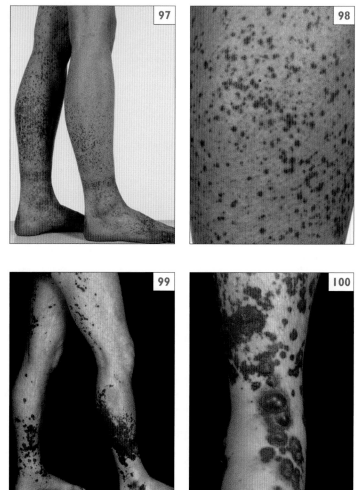

- Hepatitis B and C serology (HBV and HCV infection is associated with mixed essential cryoglobulinaemia; HBV infection is associated with systemic polyarteritis nodosa).
- HIV serology (if indicated).
- Chest radiography (alveolar haemorrhage in microscopic polyangiitis).

- Skin biopsy for histopathology (fibrinoid necrosis and leucocytoclastic vasculitis in dermal vessels is common to all causes of SVV).
- Skin biopsy for direct immuno-fluorescence (HSP may be identified by vascular luminal deposition of IgA).

IMMEDIATE MANAGEMENT

Assess the patient for systemic vasculitis: evidence of renal, neurological, or other systemic activity necessitates urgent referral to the relevant specialist. If the vasculitis is triggered by a drug, stop the culprit medication.

Topical therapy

- Bed rest and leg elevation are important first-line measures.
- Corticosteroid ointment, twice per day (use for a restricted period):
    legs and arms: potent.
- Gentle compression bandaging of the legs, if tolerated, may assist resolution.
- Ulcerated areas should be covered with nonadhesive dressings.

Systemic therapy

- Appropriate analgesia.
- If a bacterial septicaemia is suspected (e.g. meningococcal) give IV cefotaxime 1 g twice per day or benzylpenicillin 2.4 g every 4 hr.
- Once an infection has been excluded, give oral corticosteroids if purpura continues to develop (e.g. prednisolone 0.5 mg/kg/day, and reduce with response).

LONG-TERM MANAGEMENT ISSUES

In some cases an obvious trigger or associated disorder cannot be identified. In these cases development of vasculitic lesions may continue for several months. Relapsing idiopathic cutaneous SVV often responds to dapsone 50–100 mg once daily. In severe cases immunosuppressants, such as cyclophosphamide, may be necessary. Compression hosiery may also be beneficial in reducing the severity or frequency of flare-ups.

Polyarteritis nodosa

Polyarteritis nodosa (PAN) is a rare, necrotizing vasculitis affecting medium- and small-sized arteries. Skin lesions are seen in approximately 40% of patients with systemic PAN, while in cutaneous PAN, a distinct variant, vascular inflammation is limited to the skin, with only mild constitutional features and a benign course. Nodules are a typical feature of PAN but are also encountered in skin involvement in microscopic polyangiitis, Churg–Strauss syndrome, and Wegener's granulomatosis. Systemic PAN can be associated with hepatitis B infection, systemic lupus erythematosus, and inflammatory bowel disease.

CLINICAL FEATURES

The primary skin lesions in PAN are subcutaneous nodules usually found on the lower legs. The nodules are painful, tender, and may become ulcerated. Livedo reticularis on the legs is present (**101, 102**). Other cutaneous features of PAN include palpable purpura, digital gangrene, lower leg ulceration, and widespread cutaneous necrosis.

DIFFERENTIAL DIAGNOSIS

- Other vasculitides (e.g. microscopic polyangiitis, Churg–Strauss syndrome).
- Erythema nodosum (p. 100, tender, bruise-like nodules on lower legs).
- Nodular vasculitis (multiple, deep nodules on the lower legs which may ulcerate).

COMPLICATIONS

Systemic PAN:
- General: fever, arthralgia, headache, myalgia, weight loss.
- Cardiovascular system: hypertension, myocardial infarction.
- Gastrointestinal tract/renal: abdominal pain, intestinal infarction, arterial aneurysms, renal impairment.
- Nervous system: cerebrovascular ischaemia, convulsions, peripheral neuropathy.

INVESTIGATIONS
Vasculitis screen
- Blood count (neutrophilia, thrombocytosis, and normocytic anaemia in systemic PAN).
- Basic chemistry, liver function tests (impaired renal function indicates renal vasculitis).
- ESR, CRP (inflammatory markers are raised).
- Urinalysis (haematuria and proteinuria indicate renal vasculitis).
- ANCA (p-ANCA (anti-MPO) is positive in about 10% of cases of PAN).
- ANA, complement, anti-dsDNA, -Sm, -Ro(SS-A), -La(SS-B), -RNP, antibodies (to exclude SLE).
- Hepatitis B and hepatitis C serology (hepatitis B virus infection is associated with systemic PAN).

- Skin biopsy for histopathology (inflammation of the small and medium-sized arteries in deep dermis and subcutis, the infiltrate consists of neutrophils, eosinophils, and lymphocytes; at a later stage there is luminal thrombus).
- Renal or mesenteric angiography (in systemic PAN angiography may demonstrate aneurysms, stenosis, or beaded tortuosity of the medium-sized arteries of the kidney and mesentery).

Three out of 10 criteria (American College of Rheumatology) are needed to make the diagnosis of systemic PAN. The 10 criteria are: weight loss of 4 kg or more, livedo reticularis, testicular pain, myalgia or leg weakness, mono- or poly-neuropathy, diastolic BP >90 mmHg, elevated creatinine, infection with HBV, abnormality on arteriography, biopsy-proven vasculitis of small or medium-sized artery.

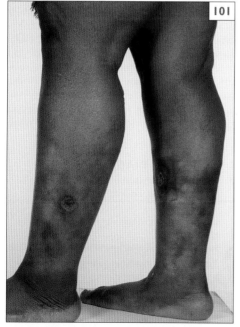

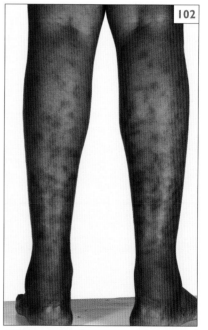

101 Cutaneous polyarteritis nodosa. There is a broken livedo reticularis on the lower legs. Several nodules were palpable, two of which had ulcerated.

102 Systemic polyarteritis nodosa. Multiple subcutaneous nodules were present and associated with a broken livedo reticularis on the lower legs. This patient also had arthritis, with involvement of the ankles.

IMMEDIATE MANAGEMENT
Systemic PAN
- Assess the patient for systemic vasculitis involvement: evidence of renal, neurological, or other systemic activity necessitates urgent referral to the relevant specialist.
- Systemic corticosteroids (e.g. prednisolone 1–2 mg/kg/day), reducing with response.

Cutaneous PAN
- Cutaneous PAN can be controlled with a short course of systemic corticosteroids (e.g. prednisolone 0.5 mg/kg/day, reducing with response).

LONG-TERM MANAGEMENT ISSUES
Cytotoxic agents, such as cyclophosphamide, are useful adjuncts to corticosteroids in systemic PAN. Compression bandaging or compression hosiery may be helpful in limiting the signs and symptoms of cutaneous PAN. Intermittent courses of prednisolone will successfully treat flares of cutaneous PAN. In chronic, symptomatic cutaneous PAN dapsone, 50–100 mg once daily, may be helpful.

Cutaneous embolism

Emboli from the heart or major arteries can become lodged in the cutaneous vasculature and cause skin ischaemia or infarction. Cholesterol emboli arise from arteriosclerotic plaques which are disturbed by arterial catheterization, other vascular manipulations (e.g. angioplasty), and anticoagulation or thrombolytic therapy for cardiac, coronary artery, or cerebrovascular disease. Fat released into the circulation following major trauma can cause cutaneous embolism. Emboli can also arise from vegetations in endocarditis and from atrial myxomas. Emboli to the skin are often accompanied by embolization of other organs which may be the cause of serious morbidity.

CLINICAL FEATURES
In cholesterol embolism the signs are usually confined to the lower extremities: there is often livedo reticularis with acral cyanosis and associated leg or foot pain. Other signs include nodules, retiform (stellate) purpura, and necrotic ulcers. In acute bacterial endocarditis well circumscribed purpuric, haemorrhagic or pustular lesions of varying size may be seen on acral skin (digits, hands, feet, nose) (**103, 104**). In subacute bacterial endocarditis micro- and macro-embolic manifestations include sub-ungual splinter haemorrhages, Osler's nodes (tender red nodules on the pulps of the fingers), and Janeway lesions (nontender, red spots on the palms and soles which blanch with compression).

DIFFERENTIAL DIAGNOSIS
- Small vessel vasculitis (p. 82, palpable purpura on dependent areas).
- Thrombophilia disorders (purpura secondary to cutaneous vascular thrombosis).
- Eccthyma gangrenosum (infection by *Pseudomonas aeruginosa* causing purpuric lesions with eschars).
- Acute arterial insufficiency (ischaemia of distal extremity).
- Other causes of widespread cutaneous necrosis (p. 88, large zones of cutaneous infarction).

103 Cutaneous embolism. A haemorrhagic infarct on the thumb of a patient with acute infective endocarditis.

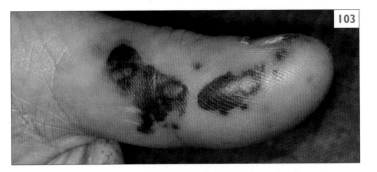

COMPLICATIONS
- Fever and malaise.
- Myalgia.
- Hypertension.
- Confusion, stroke.
- Signs of systemic emboli to kidneys, spleen, liver, gastrointestinal tract.

INVESTIGATIONS
Suspected infective endocarditis
- Blood count (anaemia, neutrophilia).
- Basic chemistry, liver function tests (impaired renal function indicates renal embolism).
- ESR, CRP (inflammatory markers will be elevated).
- Urinalysis (proteinuria, haematuria).
- Blood cultures × 3 (positive blood cultures).
- Echocardiogram (to look for vegetations).
- Skin biopsy for histopathology and microbiological culture (embolic occlusion of deep dermal vessels; emboli may be laden with bacteria; infecting organism can be cultured from septic skin embolism).

Suspected cholesterol embolism
- Blood count (eosinophilia).
- Basic chemistry, liver function tests (impaired renal function indicates renal embolism).
- Skin biopsy for histopathology from centre of blanched area within livedo reticularis (arterioles are occluded by giant cells surrounding biconvex, needle-shaped clefts corresponding to the cholesterol crystal microemboli).

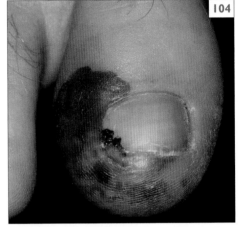

104 Cutaneous embolism. Haemorrhagic and pustular infarcts on the great toe caused by emboli arising from a cardiac valve vegetation in acute infective endocarditis.

IMMEDIATE MANAGEMENT
The diagnosis of cutaneous emboli usually indicates significant cardiac or vascular pathology and therefore an immediate referral to the appropriate specialist is necessary. In the case of acute bacterial endocarditis, intravenous antibiotics must be initiated once blood cultures have been taken. The choice of antibiotic should be guided by a microbiologist.

LONG-TERM MANAGEMENT ISSUES
Skin infarcts from emboli usually heal well once the source of emboli has been treated.

Widespread cutaneous necrosis

The term widespread cutaneous necrosis (WCN) describes extensive skin infarction caused by a range of vascular pathologies. In evaluating purpura with skin necrosis it is important to discriminate between inflammatory vascular injury (vasculitis) and noninflammatory injury (thromboembolism). The presence of retiform (or stellate) purpura points to a vaso-occlusive disorder. Multiple, large areas of skin necrosis generally indicate thrombosis within deep dermal arteries or arterioles heralding a severe systemic coagulopathy, usually disseminated intravascular coagulopathy (DIC).

CLINICAL FEATURES
WCN is characterized by large areas of purpura leading to skin necrosis. The areas of involvement are well defined and often have a branching, stellate, or retiform outline reflecting arterial occlusion (**105–107**). Signs of surrounding inflammation may be absent but blistering can occur. If full-thickness skin necrosis develops then an eschar will form. The distribution of skin necrosis can suggest the underlying aetiology; e.g. extremities in cryoglobulinaemia, breasts and buttocks in warfarin (coumarin) skin necrosis.

CAUSES OF WIDESPREAD CUTANEOUS NECROSIS
- Any cause of DIC.
- Infectious purpura fulminans (p. 130).
- Embolic infarction (p. 86).
- Anticoagulant skin necrosis (warfarin/coumarin, heparin).
- Antiphospholipid antibody syndrome (often secondary to systemic lupus erythematosus).
- Protein C/S/antithrombin disorders.
- Thrombocytosis (secondary to myeloproliferative disorder).
- Small vessel vasculitis (p. 82).
- Polyarteritis nodosa (p. 84).
- Cryoglobulinaemia, cryofibrinoginaemia.
- Calciphylaxis (p. 90).
- Necrotizing fasciitis (p. 128).
- Pyoderma gangrenosum (p. 92).
- Ecthyma (crusted and ulcerated bacterial skin infection).
- Vasculotropic fungal infection (e.g. *Mucor*).

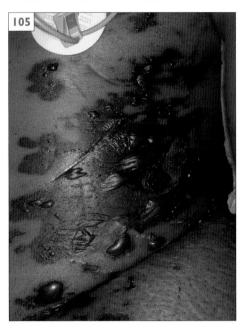

105 Widespread cutaneous necrosis. In this patient with fulminant Churg–Strauss vasculitis there is a large area of blistering skin necrosis with a retiform outline.

COMPLICATIONS
- Fever.
- Cardiovascular collapse.
- Acute renal failure.
- Multiorgan failure.

INVESTIGATIONS
Thrombophilia screen
- Blood count (severe thrombocytopenia in DIC, thrombocytosis in myeloproferative disorders).
- INR, activated partial thromboplastin time (APTT), protein C and S, antithrombin, D-dimers, fibrin degradation products (FDPs) (warfarin/coumarin skin necrosis occurs in patients deficient in protein C or S and is accompanied by a greatly prolonged INR; DIC is characterized by a prolonged PT, APTT, and thrombin time (TT), reduced fibrinogen level, high level of FDPs and D-dimers).

106 Widespread cutaneous necrosis. There are several large areas of full-thickness skin necrosis in this patient with the antiphospholipid syndrome.

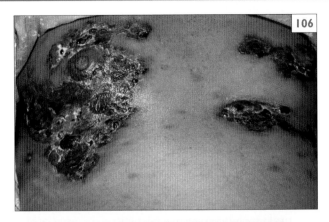

107 Widespread cutaneous necrosis. This large, stellate zone of skin necrosis occurred in a patient with DIC secondary to meningococcal septicaemia.

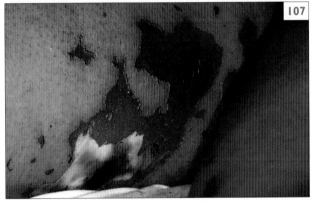

- Dilute Russell viper venom time (DRVVT), lupus anticoagulant, anticardiolipin antibodies (in the antiphospholipid syndrome DRVVT is prolonged, lupus anticoagulant and anticardiolipin antibodies are positive).
- Factor V Leiden, cryoglobulins, cryofibrinogen.
- Heparin antibodies (if relevant).
- Skin biopsy for histopathology (in DIC fibrin thrombi are present in the capillaries and venules without vasculitis or inflammation; in older lesions there is epidermal necrosis and extensive dermal haemorrhage).

Vasculitis screen

- Blood count (eosinophilia is characteristic of Churg–Strauss syndrome; neutrophilia, thrombocytosis, and normocytic anaemia occur in systemic PAN).
- Basic chemistry, liver function tests (impaired renal function indicates renal vasculitis).
- ESR, CRP (inflammatory markers are raised).
- Urinalysis (haematuria and proteinuria indicate renal vasculitis).
- ANCA (p-ANCA (anti-MPO) is positive in 60% microscopic polyangiitis and 40% Churg–Strauss syndrome; c-ANCA (anti-PR3) is positive in 90% Wegener's granulomatosis and 30% microscopic polyangiitis).
- ANA, complement, anti-dsDNA, -Sm, -Ro(SS-A), -La(SS-B), -RNP, antibodies (to exclude systemic lupus erythematosus).
- Rheumatoid factor (raised in rheumatoid arthritis and mixed essential cryoglobulinaemia).

- Cryoglobulins (raised in cryoglobulinaemia).
- Throat swab, ASOT, blood cultures (Henoch–Schönlein purpura can be triggered by an upper respiratory tract infection).
- Hepatitis B and C serology (hepatitis B virus and hepatitis C virus infection is associated with mixed essential cryoglobulinaemia; hepatitis B virus infection is associated with systemic PAN).
- HIV serology (if indicated).
- Skin biopsy for histopathology (fibrinoid necrosis and leucocytoclastic vasculitis in dermal vessels in small vessel vasculitis; inflammation of the small and medium-sized arteries in deep dermis and subcutis in PAN).

IMMEDIATE MANAGEMENT

- Patients with WCN are often critically ill. If so, admit to intensive care unit for close monitoring and cardiovascular, respiratory, metabolic, and haematological support.
- If meningococcal septicaemia is suspected (or other bacterial causes of purpura fulminans) give IV cefotaxime 1 g twice per day.
- If DIC is present give platelet transfusions and fresh frozen plasma. In infectious purpura fulminans consider infusion of recombinant human activated protein C.
- Every effort must be made to clarify the pathological processes leading to WCN. Identification of the underlying diagnosis will direct further treatment.

LONG-TERM MANAGEMENT ISSUES

Once the eschar has separated the resulting ulcers will usually heal by secondary intention. Occasionally skin grafting is required.

Calciphylaxis

Calciphylaxis is a cutaneous necrosis syndrome caused by calcification of deep dermal vessels resulting in infarction of skin and subcutis (it is also known as the vascular calcification–cutaneous necrosis syndrome, and calcific uraemic arteriolopathy). Calciphylaxis is most commonly seen in patients with end-stage renal failure and secondary hyperparathyroidism (**108**). However it can occur in patients with renal failure and a normal calcium–phosphorus product or, rarely, in patients with normal renal function. It is associated with a poor prognosis and carries a mortality rate of up to 60%.

CLINICAL FEATURES

The lesions present as painful, violaceous, reticulate areas, commonly on the thighs (**109, 110**). Palpation of the mottled, dusky skin reveals hard subcutaneous nodules and plaques. Subsequently skin necrosis develops to produce an ischaemic ulcer with associated eschar. The lesions are usually progressive, extending with purpuric, indurated margins.

DIFFERENTIAL DIAGNOSIS

- Vasculitic ulcer (punched-out ulcer within area of purpura).
- Necrotizing fasciitis (p. 128, necrotizing infection of subcutaneous tissues).
- Panniculitis (p. 102, deep-seated plaques of subcutaneous fat inflammation).
- Pyoderma grangrenosum (p. 92, painful ulcer with a necrotic base and violaceous margin).
- Other causes of widespread skin necrosis (p. 88, large zones of cutaneous infarction).

COMPLICATIONS

- Secondary bacterial infection (may lead to septicaemia).
- Gangrene.
- Multiorgan failure.

INVESTIGATIONS
- Blood count (anaemia of renal failure).
- Basic chemistry, liver function tests (elevated creatinine and urea).
- Calcium and phosphate, parathyroid hormone (elevated calcium, phosphate, and parathyroid hormone).
- Plain radiograph of thighs (extensive vascular calcification).
- Deep skin biopsy for histopathology (vascular wall calcification in medium-sized deep dermal and subcuticular arteries; there is often lobular panniculitis but no vasculitis).

IMMEDIATE MANAGEMENT
Topical therapy
- Nonadhesive dressings.
- Surgical debridement of necrotic tissue.

Systemic therapy
- Restore calcium and electrolyte levels.
- Give adequate analgesia.
- Treat any associated infection with intravenous antibiotics.
- Infusions of sodium thiosulfate can be helpful.
- Partial parathyroidectomy should be considered early to correct the hyperparathyroidism.

LONG-TERM MANAGEMENT ISSUES
Involvement of the trunk by calciphylaxis is a poor prognostic feature. On-going supportive care is essential and includes wound care, control of the renal failure, and aggressive treatment of any secondary infection.

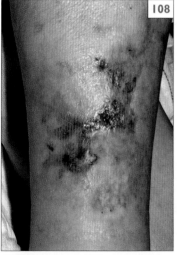

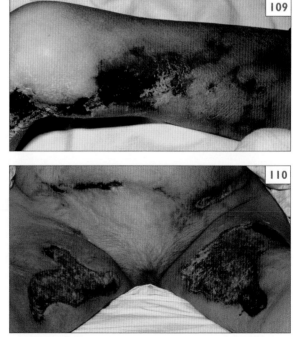

108 Calciphylaxis. This patient with end-stage renal failure and secondary hyperparathyroidism has developed calciphylaxis. There is an area of retiform skin necrosis on the shin.

109 Calciphylaxis. Extensive and full-thickness linear skin necrosis has occurred on the thigh in this patient with calciphylaxis. The necrosis has a retiform outline.

110 Calciphylaxis. Large areas of skin necrosis on the thighs have been surgically debrided. Calciphylaxis has also caused linear ulcers on the abdominal skin.

Pyoderma gangrenosum

Pyoderma grangrenosum (PG) is not primarily a vascular disorder although vasculitis-type changes may be seen histologically. The intense neutrophilic inflammation in PG induces skin destruction which usually presents as a painful, necrotic ulcer. Approximately 50% of PG cases are associated with an underlying systemic disease: inflammatory bowel disease, rheumatoid or seronegative arthritis, or haematological malignancy (myeloid leukaemias and multiple myeloma, in particular).

CLINICAL FEATURES

The fully developed lesion of PG is a painful ulcer with a necrotic base and a ragged, undermined, purple margin (**111, 112**). However, PG may begin as a nodule or haemorrhagic pustule. Beyond the dusky margin the surrounding skin is red and indurated. PG may either evolve rapidly causing widespread tissue destruction, or display a relatively indolent course. Recognized variants are bullous, pustular, and superficial granulomatous forms. Provocation of PG at the site of skin trauma occurs in 20% of cases and is termed pathergy (**113**). In these patients mistaken surgical attempts to debride the lesion can exacerbate the PG and lead to greater tissue destruction.

DIFFERENTIAL DIAGNOSIS

- Venous ulcer (indolent ulcer on lower leg, usual medial aspect).
- Arterial ulcer (punched-out ulcer on foot or lower leg).
- Vasculitic ulcer (punched-out ulcer within area of purpura).
- Necrotizing fasciitis (p. 128, necrotizing infection of subcutaneous tissues).
- Ecthyma (crusted and ulcerating bacterial skin infection).
- Panniculitis (p. 102, deep-seated plaques of subcutaneous fat inflammation).
- Calciphylaxis (p. 90, indurated, necrotizing nodules on legs in chronic renal failure patients).

COMPLICATIONS

- Secondary bacterial infection (may lead to septicaemia).

INVESTIGATIONS

- Blood count (anaemia, neutrophilia).
- Blood film (to exclude leukaemia).
- Basic chemistry, liver function tests.
- ESR (ESR usually very high).
- Rheumatoid factor (to exclude rheumatoid arthritis).
- Immunoglobulins and serum protein electrophoresis, Bence–Jones proteins (to exclude multiple myeloma).
- Other investigations to exclude inflammatory bowel disease, arthritis, and haematological malignancy (e.g. gastrointestinal endoscopy and biopsy, faecal calprotectin; joint radiography; bone marrow biopsy).
- Skin biopsy for histopathology (neutrophilic inflammation with abscess formation but no organisms; a lymphocytic or leucocytoclastic vasculitis is sometimes also seen).

IMMEDIATE MANAGEMENT
Topical therapy

- Corticosteroid ointment under dressings (use for restricted period):
     leg: potent or superpotent.
- Nonadhesive dressing.
- Gentle compression bandaging, if tolerated.

Systemic therapy

- High-dose oral corticosteroids (e.g. prednisolone 1–2 mg/kg/day), reducing with response.
- Adequate analgesia (often opiates are required).

LONG-TERM MANAGEMENT ISSUES

Once the diagnosis of PG has been made investigations should be directed to identify an associated systemic disease (see above). Any underlying disorder needs to be treated. For recalcitrant PG alternative immunosuppressants may be necessary, including ciclosporin (3–5 mg/kg/day), intravenous pulses of methylprednisolone (0.5–1 g given over 3 hr for 3 consecutive days), or intravenous immunoglobulin (1 g/kg/day for 2 consecutive days, repeatedly monthly for 3 consecutive months). An antiTNF biologic agent (e.g infliximab) may be indicated if other systemic agents are found to be ineffective or poorly tolerated.

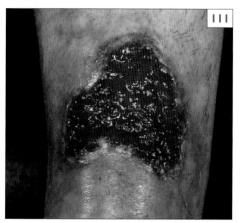

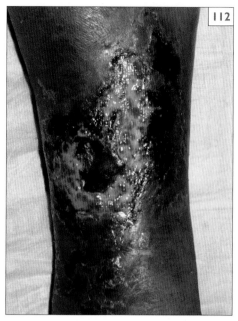

111 Pyoderma gangrenosum. There is a deep necrotic ulcer on the calf with dusky, overhanging margins. This patient had leukaemia.

112 Pyoderma gangrenosum. There is a necrotic margin to this rapidly expanding ulcer. The patient had rheumatoid arthritis.

113 Pyoderma gangrenosum. This shallow, ulcerated lesion at the wrist with blistering margins is superficial pyoderma gangrenosum. It arose at the site of vascular cannulation (an example of pathergy).

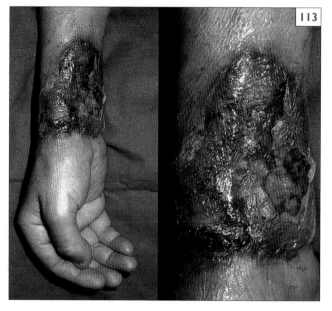

Sweet's syndrome

Sweet's syndrome (also known as acute febrile neutrophilic dermatosis) is not primarily a vascular disorder although vasculitis-type changes may be seen histologically. Intense neutrophilic inflammation of the skin is characteristic, which produces a striking eruption often accompanied by a number of systemic features. Approximately one-half of cases are associated with an underlying disorder; in 20% this is a haematological malignancy (acute myelomonocytic leukaemia, in particular). Sweet's syndrome may also be associated with inflammatory bowel disease and certain infections (e.g. *Chlamydia*, *Streptococcus*). There is a female preponderance. A Sweet's-like eruption can be triggered by the administration of granulocyte-colony stimulating factor.

CLINICAL FEATURES
Painful red papules appear which rapidly develop into deep red plaques (**114**). The eruption favours the head, neck, and upper limbs, but can occur anywhere. Lesions tend to be quite large, measuring 2–5 cm in diameter (**115**) and can be few in number or multiple. Initially the lesions have a smooth surface but, with time, can become pseudovesicular. The patient often has a fever as the lesions appear and may experience a variety of other constitutional symptoms (see below).

DIFFERENTIAL DIAGNOSIS
- Erysipelas/cellulitis (p. 126, zone of painful, spreading erythema with fever).
- Insect bites (p. 164, itchy, grouped papules or nodules).
- Urticarial vasculitis (p. 62, itchy or burning weals which are persistent).
- Cutaneous lymphoma/leukaemia cutis (p. 198, firm, red nodule or plaque).

COMPLICATIONS
- Fever.
- Arthralgia and myalgia.
- Conjunctivitis and uveitis.
- Neutrophilic alveolitis.
- Renal impairment.

INVESTIGATIONS
- Blood count and film (neutrophilia).
- Basic chemistry, liver function tests.
- ESR, CRP (inflammatory markers are elevated).
- Streptococcal and chlamydial serology.
- Immunoglobulins and serum protein electrophoresis, Bence–Jones proteins (to exclude multiple myeloma).
- Other investigations to exclude inflammatory bowel disease and haematological malignancy (e.g. gastrointestinal endoscopy and biopsy, faecal calprotectin; joint radiography; bone marrow biopsy).
- Skin biopsy for histopathology (upper dermal oedema, a dense neutrophilic infiltrate in the mid-dermis, neutrophils aggregate around vessels, but usually without overt vasculitis).

IMMEDIATE MANAGEMENT
Topical therapy
- Corticosteroid ointment, twice per day (use for restricted period):
    face: moderately potent.
    trunk, limbs: potent or superpotent.

Systemic therapy
- Oral corticosteroids (e.g. prednisolone 0.5–1 mg/kg/day), reducing with response.

LONG-TERM MANAGEMENT ISSUES
Investigations should be directed to a search for a systemic disease associated with Sweet's syndrome. Untreated, the lesions enlarge but eventually resolve without scarring over several weeks. With systemic corticosteroids, the lesions usually resolve within a few days. In patients with recalcitrant Sweet's syndrome other agents which can be used alone or in combination with oral corticosteroids include dapsone and colchicine. Recurrences occur in approximately 50% of patients.

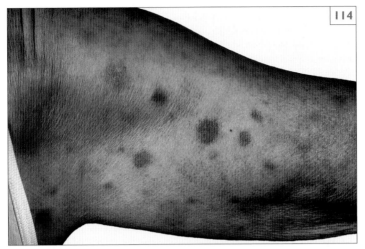

114 Sweet's syndrome. There are multiple, deep red nodules and small plaques on the arms of this patient with myelodysplasia.

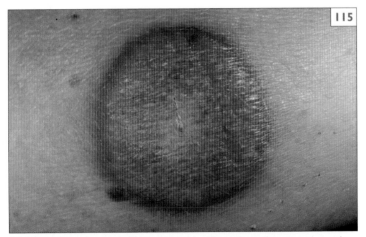

115 Sweet's syndrome. Individual lesions of Sweet's syndrome are round and and measure 2–5 cm in diameter. The surface is usually smooth.

Dependency syndrome

The dependency syndrome generally occurs in elderly patients who have poor mobility, are largely chair-bound, and may be overweight. The patient often sleeps in their chair at night. Swelling and redness of the lower legs, characteristic of the dependency syndrome, is caused by a combination of sustained venous downforce, producing venous insufficiency, and persistent lymphatic overload, causing lymphoedema. Although the dependency syndrome is a complication of chronic mobility problems the skin redness can develop suddenly and be mistaken for cellulitis or DVT. The same clinical features can be caused by a large pelvic mass compressing proximal veins and lymphatics.

CLINICAL FEATURES

The physical signs in the lower limbs are usually symmetrical and are often accompanied by itching or pain. There is demonstrable pitting oedema as well as fixed swelling (lymphoedema) of the lower legs and feet (**116, 117**). Chronic swelling will result in a 'cobblestone' appearance of the skin of the shins with deep creases at the ankles and toes. If arterial perfusion is poor the toes may be dusky. Large blisters may occur if accumulation of oedema has been rapid. The shins and calves are red and may be warm on palpation. Venous eczema is also often present which, if untreated, may become hyperkeratotic. There may be other signs of venous insufficiency, e.g. varicose veins, lipodermatosclerosis, venous ulceration. Secondary superficial bacterial infection with *Staphylococcus* or *Streptococcus* is common and may lead to cellulitis.

DIFFERENTIAL DIAGNOSIS

- Venous eczema (p. 16, eczema on lower legs caused by venous insufficiency).
- Lymphoedema (nonpitting oedema with textural changes to the skin).
- Allergic contact dermatitis (p. 18, eczema in localized area or unusual distribution).
- Deep venous thrombosis (limb swelling, erythema, and pain).
- Erysipelas/cellulitis (p. 126, zone of painful, spreading erythema with fever).
- Bullous pemphigoid (p. 66, itchy erythema with large tense blisters).

COMPLICATIONS

- Erysipelas/cellulitis.

INVESTIGATIONS

The diagnosis is made clinically, but the following investigations may be helpful in management:

- Skin swabs (to exclude bacterial infection).
- Ankle–brachial pressure index (to assess the capacity of distal arteries to tolerate compression).
- Venous studies (to identify a reversible cause of venous incompetence).

IMMEDIATE MANAGEMENT
Topical therapy

- General emollient therapy.
- Corticosteroid ointment, twice per day (use for restricted period):
    legs: moderately potent or potent.
- A topical steroid containing an antibiotic may be indicated if there is secondary superficial infection.
- Oedema blisters should be decompressed and covered with nonadhesive dressings.
- Advise patient to keep legs elevated when sitting and to sleep in a bed at night.
- If arterial function is adequate, gentle compression bandaging from the fore-foot to below the knee will reduce the swelling and erythema. The bandaging must be reviewed after 24 hr, initially, to ensure that peripheral perfusion has not been compromised.

Systemic therapy

- If there is significant skin infection, oral or intravenous antibiotics are indicated.

LONG-TERM MANAGEMENT ISSUES

Once the swelling and redness has been reduced by leg elevation and compression bandaging, the patient should be encouraged to wear class 1 or 2, below-knee, compression hosiery. Management from the general physicians must be directed to improving mobility by treating any associated arthritic or cardiopulmonary problems. Particular attention must be paid to managing other causes of peripheral oedema, such as hypoalbuminaemia and right-sided heart failure. Some patients may benefit from weight reduction.

116 Dependency syndrome. This woman's legs show the signs of both lymphoedema (swelling, deep creases at the ankles) and venous congestion (erythema and eczematous changes).

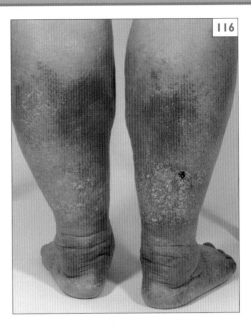

117 Dependency syndrome. This elderly man with chronic pulmonary disease was unable to lie flat and had slept in a chair for many months. Longstanding immobility and dependency has lead to swollen, red legs.

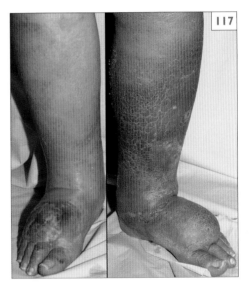

CHAPTER 8

Panniculitis

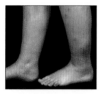

Erythema nodosum

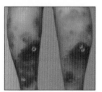

Panniculitis

Erythema nodosum

Erythema nodosum (EN) is a form of panniculitis (inflammation of the subcutaneous fat) with a characteristic clinical presentation. The incidence peaks between the second and fourth decades and is more common in women. EN generally occurs as a reaction to an underlying disorder. The associations are: inflammatory diseases (sarcoidosis, inflammatory bowel disease, Behcet's disease); bacterial infections (*Streptococcus*, TB, *Chlamydia*); viral infections (infectious mononucleosis, hepatitis B); fungal and protozoal infections (toxoplasmosis, amoebiasis); drugs (sulphonamides, oral contraceptive pill); neoplasms (lymphoma, renal cell carcinoma).

CLINICAL FEATURES
Painful, red nodules and plaques appear on the lower legs, particularly over the shins (**118**). Lesions are usually relatively few in number, between one and six, and vary between 2 and 5 cm in diameter. On palpation they are smooth, indurated, warm, and tender; often the clinical features are best appreciated by palpation. The lesions change colour over 3–4 weeks from red to purple and then fade, like a bruise. In darkly pigmented skin EN lesions can be hyperpigmented (**119**). Rarely, EN can appear at sites other than the lower legs.

DIFFERENTIAL DIAGNOSIS
- Other forms of panniculitis (p. 102, red, painful plaques, may ulcerate).
- Erysipelas/cellulitis (p. 126, zone of painful, spreading erythema with fever).
- Polyarteritis nodosa (p. 84, subcutaneous nodules on the lower legs with livedo reticularis).
- Nodular vasculitis (multiple, deep nodules on the lower legs which may ulcerate).
- Calciphylaxis (p. 90, indurated, necrotizing nodules on the legs in chronic renal failure patients).

COMPLICATIONS
- Fever and malaise.
- Arthralgia.
- Headache.
- Abdominal pain, diarrhoea, vomiting.

INVESTIGATIONS
- Blood count, basic chemistry, liver function tests (useful as indicators of general health and associated systemic cause).
- ESR, CRP (raised).
- Investigations for specific cause:
- Streptococcal serology.
- Hepatitis B serology.
- EBV serology.
- Serum ACE.
- Chest radiography.
- Mantoux test.
- Faecal calprotectin.
- Deep skin biopsy for histopathology (panniculitis which is predominantly septal; the superficial and deep inflammatory infiltrate is perivascular and often extends into the dermis).

IMMEDIATE MANAGEMENT
Topical therapy
- Leg elevation, preferably as bed rest.
- Gentle leg compression with elasticated, tubular bandages.

Systemic therapy
- Adequate analgesia.
- Treatment should be directed to managing the underlying disorder.
- If an infective trigger has been excluded or treated then oral corticosteroids can be given to settle symptomatic EN (e.g. prednisolone 20–30 mg daily reducing with response).

LONG-TERM MANAGEMENT ISSUES
In some patients an underlying cause cannot be found. If these patients are developing recurrent EN, acute relapses can be treated with a short course of oral steroids. However if the EN is becoming chronic, dapsone 50–100 mg once daily can be used to induce a remission. Compression hosiery is also useful.

118 Erythema nodosum. Bruise-like, tender nodules on the legs of a patient with active ulcerative colitis.

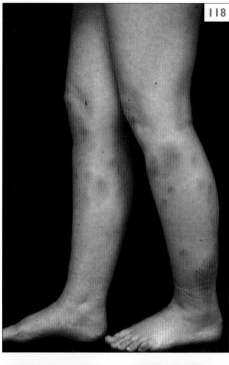

119 Erythema nodosum. In dark skin the lesions of erythema nodosum can be hyperpigmented.

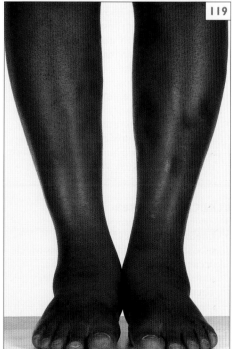

Panniculitis

The panniculitides are a group of dermatoses characterized by inflammation of the subcutaneous fat. There is a range of aetiologies and in each case investigations must be directed to identifying the cause and any relevant systemic association. The clinical appearance of panniculitis is similar for all causes. The subtypes of panniculitis are:

- Erythema nodosum: usually occurs as a reaction to a systemic inflammatory or infective illness (see p. 100).
- Lupus panniculitis (lupus profundus): an uncommon form of cutaneous lupus erythematosus.
- Pancreatic panniculitis: a complication of pancreatic disease (e.g. pancreatitis or carcinoma).
- Alpha-1-antitrypsin deficiency panniculitis: occurs in patients with very low levels of alpha-1-antitrypsin.
- Infectious panniculitis: infection of subcutis via direct inoculation or septicaemia. Patients are often immunocompromised.
- Chemical/foreign body panniculitis: due to the injection of substances into the subcutaneous fat. It may be a manifestation of dermatitis artefacta (factitial panniculitis).
- Lipodermatosclerosis: occurs on the lower legs secondary to chronic venous insufficiency.
- Subcutaneous panniculitis-like T cell lymphoma: a cytotoxic T cell lymphoma which preferentially infiltrates the subcutis. It is often associated with haemophagocytic activity.

CLINICAL FEATURES

- Erythema nodosum: see p. 100.
- Lupus panniculitis (**120**): tender, subcutaneous nodules and plaques which occur on the face, upper outer arms, shoulders, hips, trunk, and lower legs. There is sometimes a history of precipitating trauma. Lesions evolve with lipoatrophy to produce deep depressions.
- Pancreatic panniculitis (**121**): multiple, red, subcutaneous nodules on the legs which become fluctuant and ulcerate, discharging a brown oily material.
- Alpha-1-antitrypsin deficiency panniculitis (**122**): painful, red–purple subcutaneous nodules and plaques on flanks, buttocks, and thighs which may ulcerate to produce an oily exudate.
- Infectious panniculitis: red nodules and plaques which may become fluctuant, ulcerate, and produce a purulent discharge.
- Chemical/foreign body panniculitis: red, subcutaneous nodules and plaques at sites easily reached, such as thighs and abdomen.
- Lipodermatosclerosis: there is a zone of erythema and induration, usually occurring on the medial aspect of the lower leg. Over time sclerosis, hyperpigmentation, and circumferential sclerosis occur, producing the contour of an inverted wine bottle.

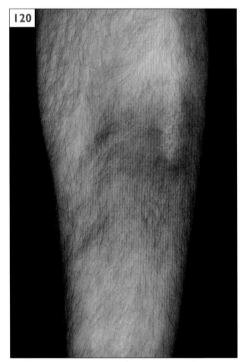

120 Panniculitis. There is a large zone of erythema on the shin which was warm and indurated on palpation. The patient had systemic lupus erythematosus and lupus profundus.

121 Panniculitis. Ulcerated panniculitis with an oily discharge in a patient with chronic pancreatitis.

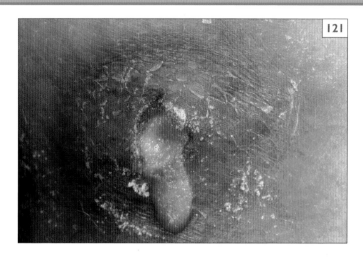

- Subcutaneous panniculitis-like T cell lymphoma: painful, red or purpuric subcutaneous nodules and plaques on arms, legs, and trunk.

DIFFERENTIAL DIAGNOSIS
- Erysipelas/cellulitis (p. 126, zone of painful, spreading erythema with fever).
- Polyarteritis nodosa (p. 84, subcutaneous nodules on the lower legs with livedo reticularis).
- Nodular vasculitis (multiple, deep nodules on the lower legs which may ulcerate).
- Calciphylaxis (p. 90, indurated, necrotizing nodules on legs in chronic renal failure patients).

COMPLICATIONS
- Fever and malaise.
- Arthralgia.

INVESTIGATIONS
- Blood count, basic chemistry, liver function tests (useful as indicators of general health and associated systemic cause).
- ESR, CRP (raised).
- Lactate dehydrogenase (LDH) (may be raised in T cell lymphoma).
- Amylase (raised in pancreatitis or pancreatic carcinoma).
- ANA, complement, anti-dsDNA, -Sm, -Ro(SS-A), -La(SS-B) (if SLE is suspected).

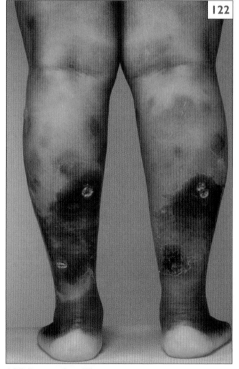

122 Panniculitis. There are numerous hyperpigmented, inflammatory plaques on the lower legs, some of which have ulcerated. The patient had alpha-1-antitrypsin deficiency.

- Alpha-1-antitrypsin (reduced in deficiency state).
- Deep skin biopsy for histopathology and culture:
- Erythema nodosum: see p. 100.
- Lupus panniculitis: lobular panniculitis with hyalin necrosis and a lymphoplasmocytic infiltrate.
- Pancreatic panniculitis: neutrophilic inflammation, cellular necrosis, and deposition of homogeneous basophilic material (due to saponification of fat by calcium salts).
- Alpha-1-antitrypsin deficiency panniculitis: neutrophilic panniculitis with necrosis and destruction of fat lobules.
- Infectious panniculitis: mixed septal/lobular panniculitis with neutrophilic infiltration, haemorrhage, and necrosis. Organisms are seen with special stains.
- Chemical/foreign body panniculitis: mostly a lobular panniculitis with neutrophilic infiltrate in early lesions and granulomatous inflammation in later lesions. Foreign material may be identified by examination under polarized light.
- Lipodermatosclerosis: lymphocytic infiltrate, capillary congestion, lobular ischaemia, lipomembranous (membranocystic) fat necrosis.
- Subcutaneous panniculitis-like T cell lymphoma: mixed septal and lobular panniculitis with foci of fat necrosis. Atypical lymphoid cells may be present. Enlarged macrophages may contain other ingested cells or cell fragments ('bean bag cells' of cytophagic activity). Sample sent for T cell receptor gene rearrangement studies demonstrates a clone.

IMMEDIATE MANAGEMENT

Direct investigations to identify the underlying cause.

- Erythema nodosum: oral corticosteroids (e.g. prednisolone 20–30 mg daily reducing with response).
- Lupus panniculitis: hydroxychloroquine 200 mg once or twice daily (or 6.5 mg/kg/day). Intralesional corticosteroid injections. If very active use oral corticosteroids (e.g. prednisolone 0.5–1 mg/kg daily reducing with response).
- Pancreatic panniculitis: treat pancreatic disease.
- Alpha-1-antitrypsin deficiency panniculitis: alpha-1-antitrypsin infusions 60 mg/kg/week administered over 3–7 weeks.
- Infectious panniculitis: intravenous antibiotics, guided by microbiological advice.
- Chemical/foreign body panniculitis: stop injection of foreign material.
- Lipodermatosclerosis: compression, initially with bandages and then elasticated hosiery.
- Subcutaneous panniculitis-like T cell lymphoma: oral corticosteroids (e.g. prednisolone 0.5–1 mg/kg daily reducing with response). CHOP chemotherapy (cyclophosphamide, doxorubicin, vincristine, prednisolone).

LONG-TERM MANAGEMENT ISSUES

Long-term therapy and prognosis will depend on the underlying cause. Once panniculitis has resolved there is often a significant, disfiguring textural deficit which, if on the face, may require reconstructive surgical intervention.

Connective tissue diseases

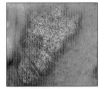 **Discoid lupus erythematosus**

 Systemic lupus erythematosus

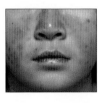 **Subacute cutaneous lupus erythematosus**

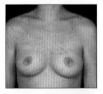 **Adult-onset Still's disease**

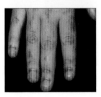 **Dermatomyositis**

Discoid lupus erythematosus

Discoid lupus erythematosus (DLE) is an autoimmune disorder characterized by inflammatory skin lesions which are often exacerbated by sunlight. Women tend to be affected more than men with a usual age of onset from 20–45 years. Thirty percent of patients with systemic lupus erythematosus will develop DLE. The lesions of DLE often occur on the face and usually prompt the patient to seek an urgent opinion.

CLINICAL FEATURES

In DLE well defined, indurated, red plaques occur on the cheeks, forehead, nose, ears (preauricular involvement is common) (**123**), and scalp. There is surface scaling and plugging of follicles by keratin. In the concha of the ears there are prominent follicular pits which are plugged with scale. In dark-skinned patients lesions may display central depigmentation and hyperpigmentation at the margins

(**124**). Lesions tend to heal with scarring which can cause permanent hair loss if the scalp is affected. Active DLE is characterized by expansion of pre-existing lesions and the development of new lupus plaques. Disseminated DLE generally occurs in women and carries a greater risk of developing into systemic lupus erythematosus (**125**).

DIFFERENTIAL DIAGNOSIS
On face and torso
- Plaque psoriasis (p. 28, scaly plaques distributed symmetrically, typical nail changes).
- Tinea facei (p. 154, annular lesion(s) with inflammatory margin).
- Lichen planus (p. 36, violaceous papules and plaques, typical changes in mouth).
- Bowen's disease (intraepidermal carcinoma: red patch with mild scale and distinct margin).
- Solar keratosis (intraepidermal dysplasia: small, scaly, red patches, often multiple).

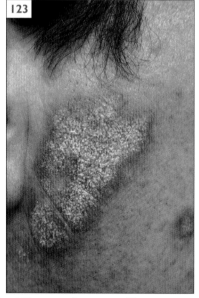

123 Discoid lupus erythematosus. The preauricular skin is a common site for DLE. This plaque shows prominent follicular plugging.

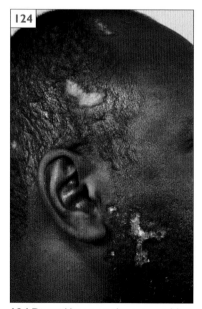

124 Discoid lupus erythematosus. Numerous lesions on the face and scalp causing scarring hair loss. In dark skin, established DLE often has a hyperpigmented margin and a depigmented centre.

On scalp
- Tinea capitis (p. 154, scaly, inflammatory patches with hair loss).
- Sarcoid (p. 46, nonscaly, violaceous plaques causing scarring alopecia).
- Lichen planus (p. 36, violaceous patches causing scarring alopecia).
- Alopecia areata (autoimmune hair loss: nonscarring patches of alopecia).

COMPLICATIONS
There are usually none.

INVESTIGATIONS
- Skin biopsy for histopathology (lymphocytic infiltrate at the dermoepidermal junction with basal keratinocyte degeneration; similar inflammation of adnexal structures, e.g. hair follicles).
- Skin biopsy for direct immunofluorescence (granular deposition of IgG and IgM at the dermoepidermal junction).
- ANA, complement, anti-dsDNA, -Sm, -RNP, -Ro(SS-A), -La(SS-B) antibodies (if SLE is suspected).

- Blood count, basic chemistry, liver function tests, ESR, urinalysis (if systemic lupus erythematosus is suspected and as baseline for monitoring of systemic therapy).

IMMEDIATE MANAGEMENT
Topical therapy
- Corticosteroid ointment, twice per day (use for a restricted period):
    face and scalp: potent or superpotent.
    trunk and limbs: superpotent.
- Photoprotection: broad-spectrum topical sunscreen and a wide-brimmed hat.
- The patient should be advised against excessive sunlight avoidance.

Systemic therapy
- In extensive DLE a course of oral corticosteroid can be helpful (e.g. prednisolone 0.5 mg/kg/day for 1 week, thereafter reduced by 5 mg every 5 days).

LONG-TERM MANAGEMENT ISSUES
Since DLE lesions heal with scarring, aggressive corticosteroid topical therapy is appropriate. Patients who fail to respond to topical treatment may improve with hydroxychloroquine 200 mg once or twice daily (or 6.5 mg/kg/day). If hydroxychloroquine is unsuccessful, consider acitretin. Patients who suffer intermittent DLE flares need to be under regular follow-up by a dermatologist so that therapy can be tailored to disease activity. In disfiguring facial DLE cosmetic camouflage make-up can be useful. Complete remission occurs in approximately 50% of patients with localized DLE. Approximately 5% of patients will develop systemic lupus erythematosus. Disseminated DLE is more persistent and has a stronger association with systemic lupus erythematosus.

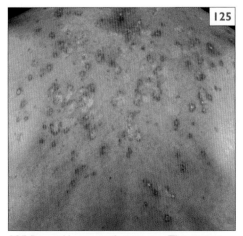

125 Discoid lupus erythematosus. This patient has disseminated DLE. There are multiple small lesions on the upper back which have red margins and hypopigmented, scarred centres.

Systemic lupus erythematosus

Systemic lupus erythematosus (SLE) is an auto-immune disease with a spectrum of clinical activity which ranges from mild to life-threatening. It affects young women more than men with an onset usually between the ages of 16 and 55 years. It is not uncommon for a patient with SLE to present acutely with a multisystem illness which includes prominent skin signs.

CLINICAL FEATURES

The usual rash of SLE is a well defined erythema involving the cheeks and bridge of the nose (butterfly rash) (**126**). The eruption is photosensitive and may occur in association with macular erythema on other sun-exposed sites (e.g. ears, neck, V of chest, upper back, arms, and hands). In cases of acute onset the rash may blister and desquamate (**127**). Examination of the hands usually reveals nail fold erythema and visible dilated capillaries as well as ragged cuticles (**128**). There may also be a reticulate telangiectatic erythema on the palms and fingers and perniotic lesions on the finger tips or toes (chilblain lupus). A history of Raynaud's phenomenon is usual. Livedo reticularis on the legs and arms occurs commonly (**129**). Other cutaneous signs in SLE include: DLE, diffuse nonscarring alopecia, mouth ulcers, palpable purpura, and urticarial vasculitis.

DIFFERENTIAL DIAGNOSIS

- Rosacea (papules, pustules, telangiectasiae, and erythema on the face).
- Seborrhoeic dermatitis (p. 20, erythema and scaling of the face, scalp, and chest).
- Polymorphic light eruption (p. 208, itchy papules on uncovered sites developing hours after sun exposure).
- Phototoxic drug eruption (p. 222, eruption on exposed skin triggered by a photosensitizing drug).
- Dermatomyositis (p. 114, violaceous eyelid erythema, Gottron's papules, and myopathy).
- Subacute cutaneous lupus erythematosus (p. 110, annular and polycyclic eruption on upper torso).
- Mixed connective tissue disease (an overlap syndrome of SLE, systemic sclerosis, and myositis).

COMPLICATIONS

- Malaise and fatigue.
- Fever.
- Weight loss.
- Serositis (pleurisy, pericarditis).
- Arthritis (Jaccoud's).
- Renal involvement (glomerulonephritis, nephrotic syndrome).
- Hypertension (accompanies renal involvement).
- Antiphospholipid syndrome.
- Myositis.
- Pulmonary fibrosis.
- Peripheral neuropathy.
- Cerebral infarcts.
- Psychosis.
- Vasculitis.

INVESTIGATIONS

- Blood count (anaemia, leucopenia, lymphopenia, and thrombocytopenia may accompany SLE).
- Basic chemistry, liver function tests (renal impairment is common, hepatic impairment is rare).
- ESR, CRP (an elevated ESR with normal CRP is typical in SLE).
- ANA, anti-dsDNA, -Sm, -RNP, -Ro(SS-A), -La(SS-B) antibodies (ANA is usually strongly positive; anti-dsDNA and Sm antibodies are specific for SLE).
- Complement (C3 and C4 may be low in active SLE; deficiencies of C1q, C4, and C2 predispose to SLE).
- Lupus anticoagulant and anticardiolipin antibodies (anticardiolipin antibodies are present in the antiphospholipid syndrome, which occurs in approximately 30% of SLE patients).
- Urinalysis (proteinuria accompanies renal disease).
- Skin biopsy for histopathology (prominent vacuolar degeneration in the basal layer of the epidermis; in the upper dermis there is oedema and a perivascular, lymphocytic infiltrate).
- Skin biopsy for direct immunofluorescence (a granular, band-like deposition of IgG, IgM, and C3 at the dermoepidermal junction).

Four out of 11 criteria (American College of Rheumatology) are needed to make the diag-

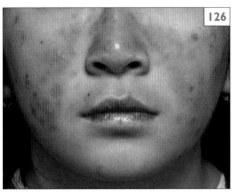

126 Systemic lupus erythematosus. There is a characteristic symmetrical erythema on the cheeks and nose (butterfly rash) in this young woman presenting with SLE.

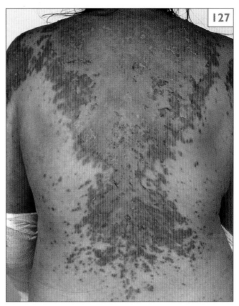

127 Systemic lupus erythematosus. This patient with acute SLE has a large zone of desquamating erythema on the back.

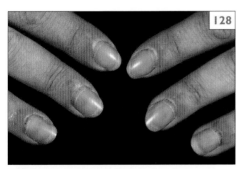

129 Systemic lupus erythematosus. Livedo reticularis is common in active SLE.

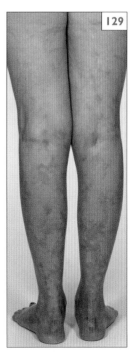

128 Systemic lupus erythematosus. There is erythema of the nail folds with dilated capillaries and ragged cuticles. Periungual erythema and nail fold changes can be seen in many connective tissue diseases.

nosis of SLE. The 11 criteria are: serositis, oral ulcers, arthritis, photosensitivity, blood disorders, renal involvement, ANA, immunological phenomena, neurological disorder, malar rash, discoid rash.

IMMEDIATE MANAGEMENT
Topical therapy
- Corticosteroid ointment, twice per day (use for a restricted period):
  - face: mildly potent.
  - trunk and limbs: potent.
- A broad-spectrum topical sunscreen should be used in conjunction with photoprotective clothing and sunlight avoidance.

Systemic therapy
- Moderate- to high-dose oral corticosteroid (e.g. prednisolone 0.5–1 mg/kg/day) reducing with response.
- In severe disease: pulsed IV methylprednisolone 500 mg for three daily doses and IV cyclophosphamide 500 mg given every 14 days for six doses.

Supportive therapy
- If acutely ill, admit to hospital for bed rest, investigations, and initiation of therapy.
- Patients with severe renal involvement will need urgent nephrology assessment.

LONG-TERM MANAGEMENT ISSUES
SLE is a relapsing–remitting disorder and treatment must be varied according to the disease activity. Many patients will require oral corticosteroid at low–moderate dosage to maintain disease control. Hydroxychloroquine 200 mg once or twice daily (or 6.5 mg/kg/day) may be used either alone or in combination with low-dose prednisolone in mild cases. Oral immunosuppressive drugs (e.g. azathioprine, cyclophosphamide, mycophenolate mofetil, methotrexate) are used as steroid-sparing agents. Prolonged use of systemic corticosteroids requires on-going screening for diabetes and hypertension and prophylaxis against osteoporosis. Gastric protection with a proton pump inhibitor is often needed (e.g. omeprazole 20 mg once daily). Patients with SLE often require management from a multidisciplinary team, including rheumatologists, nephrologists, and dermatologists.

Subacute cutaneous lupus erythematosus

Subacute cutaneous lupus erythematosus (SCLE) is a distinctive dermatosis within the spectrum of lupus erythematosus skin disease. Although it can present as an isolated disorder, the rash of SCLE may occur in the context of systemic lupus erythematosus. Certain drugs, including antihypertensives, antifungals, and anti-TNF agents, are important triggers for SCLE. There is a predilection for young, fair-skinned women. SCLE often develops acutely causing the patient to seek an urgent opinion.

CLINICAL FEATURES
The eruption of SCLE is characterized by red papules, plaques, or annular lesions on the upper chest, upper back, neck, and proximal arms (**130**). Confluence of annular lesions produces characteristic polycyclic lesions. The margins of the lesions may be scaly or become eroded (**131**). The eruption is often sore, sometimes itchy. Severe involvement may be accompanied by widespread blistering which resembles an autoimmune bullous disease or toxic epidermal necrolysis. In 50% of cases there is abnormal photosensitivity, with patients developing polymorphic light eruption or macular erythema on exposed skin. Localized areas of involvement tend to resolve leaving telangiectasiae. Other cutaneous features of SCLE include: Raynaud's phenomenon, livedo reticularis, mouth ulcers, and nonscarring alopecia.

DIFFERENTIAL DIAGNOSIS
- Plaque psoriasis (p. 28, scaly plaques distributed symmetrically, typical nail changes).
- Seborrhoeic dermatitis (p. 20, erythema and scaling of the face, scalp, and chest).
- Dermatomyositis (p. 114, violaceous eyelid erythema, Gottron's papules, and myopathy).
- Systemic lupus erythematosus (p. 108, butterfly rash, periungual erythema, and systemic features).
- Tinea corporis and facei (p. 154, asymmetrical annular lesion(s) with inflammatory margin).
- Pemphigus foliaceous (p. 68, scaly patches with blisters and erosions).

COMPLICATIONS
- Malaise and fatigue.
- Arthralgia.
- Fever.

INVESTIGATIONS
- Anti-Ro(SS-A) and -La(SS-B) antibodies (anti-Ro antibodies occur in approximately 80% and anti-La in 40% of patients with SCLE).
- Blood count, basic chemistry, liver function tests, ESR (as indicator of general health and as baseline for monitoring systemic therapy).
- ANA, complement, anti-dsDNA, -Sm, -RNP antibodies (to exclude systemic lupus erythematosus).
- Lupus anticoagulant and anticardiolipin antibodies (to exclude antiphopholipid syndrome).
- Skin biopsy for histopathology (lymphocytic infiltrate at the dermoepidermal junction with epidermal atrophy, basal vacuolar change, and apoptotic keratinocytes).
- Skin biopsy for direct immunofluorescence (granular deposition of IgG at the dermoepidermal junction).

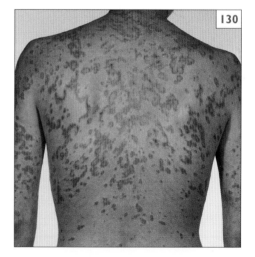

130 Subacute cutaneous lupus erythematosus. There are multiple annular, red lesions on the back which are coalescing to produce a figurate or polycyclic pattern.

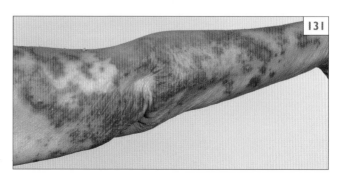

131 Subacute cutaneous lupus erythematosus. Lesional skin in SCLE often has an active, scaly margin.

IMMEDIATE MANAGEMENT
Topical therapy
- Corticosteroid ointment, twice per day (use for a restricted period):
  face: mildly potent.
  trunk and limbs: potent.
- A broad-spectrum topical sunscreen should be used in conjunction with photoprotective clothing and a wide-brimmed hat.
- The patient should be advised against excessive sunlight exposure.

Systemic therapy
- Stop any drugs which may precipitate SCLE (consider the following: calcium channel blockers, ACE inhibitors, hydrochlorothiazide, griseofulvin, terbinafine).
- In extensive SCLE a course of oral corticosteroid can be helpful (e.g. prednisolone 0.5 mg/kg/day for 1 week, thereafter reduced by 5 mg every 5 days).

LONG-TERM MANAGEMENT ISSUES
SCLE often relapses during the summer months and these patients may benefit from hydroxychloroquine 200 mg once or twice daily (or 6.5 mg/kg/day). Patients who are clearly photosensitive need to adhere to scrupulous photoprotection and sun avoidance. Systemic retinoids (e.g. acitretin) and thalidomide have also been used to control chronic, relapsing SCLE. Patients with SCLE may develop SLE and so serial monitoring of autoantibodies is recommended. Regular dermatological follow-up is usually necessary.

Adult-onset Still's disease

Adult-onset Still's disease (ASD) is a rare inflammatory condition characterized by an evanescent rash, arthritis, and spiking fevers. The eruption of ASD is a prominent part of the illness but may be absent when the patient first presents. Nonetheless, the history and associated systemic features should alert the physician to the diagnosis and prompt a review of the patient when the skin signs are active.

CLINICAL FEATURES
The fever, which is a characteristic finding in all patients, tends to occur in the late afternoon and is accompanied by myalgia, arthralgia, and a distinctive exanthem. The rash is composed of pink macules, often surrounded by pallor, which favour the trunk and limbs and may exhibit the Koebner phenomenon (**132, 133**). The rash is transient and asymptomatic, lasting only a few hours. In later stages of the disease, skin involvement may develop into a widespread, confluent, macular erythema.

DIFFERENTIAL DIAGNOSIS
- Urticaria (p. 56, itchy weals which last for less than 24 hr).
- Toxic erythema (pp. 140, 200, a widespread, morbilliform eruption of macules caused by a drug sensitivity or viral infection).
- Symptomatic dermographism (p. 60, itchy weals provoked by scratching and rubbing of the skin).
- Erythema marginatum (annular or arcuate erythema which accompanies rheumatic fever, prominent in the afternoon and lasting for a few hours).

COMPLICATIONS
- Fever (often higher than 39°C).
- Malaise.
- Arthralgia (typically wrists and cervical spine).
- Myalgia.
- Lymphadenopathy.
- Splenomegaly.
- Pericarditis.
- Pleurisy.

INVESTIGATIONS
- The diagnosis is usually made clinically.
- Blood count (anaemia of chronic disease, leucocytosis).
- Liver function tests (elevated liver enzymes can occur).
- ESR, CRP (ESR is usually elevated).
- Ferritin (often extremely high).
- Skin biopsy for histopathology (interstitial and perivascular mixed inflammatory cell infiltrate which is rich in neutrophils; there is no vasculitis).

IMMEDIATE MANAGEMENT
Topical therapy
- General emollient therapy.

Systemic therapy
- High-dose aspirin or a NSAID can help the fever and arthralgia.
- A course of oral corticosteroids can be helpful (e.g. prednisolone 0.5–1.0 mg/kg daily for 1 week, thereafter reduced by 5 mg every 7 days).

Supportive therapy
- If acutely ill, the patient should be admitted to hospital for bed rest, investigations, and initiation of therapy.

LONG-TERM MANAGEMENT ISSUES
The goals of treatment are to reduce joint inflammation and erosive synovitis. Wrist joint involvement can be followed by carpal ankylosis with decreased movement but only modest pain. Methotrexate, gold, azathioprine, and mycophenolate mofetil may all be used as steroid-sparing agents.

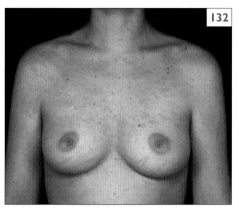

132 Adult-onset Still's disease. The eruption of pink macules is evanescent and lasts for only a few hours. Sometimes the lesions are linear reflecting Koebner's phenomenon.

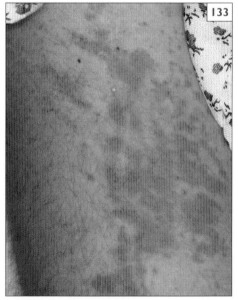

133 Adult-onset Still's disease. There are urticated, red, streaky lesions on this patient's thigh. At the time the photograph was taken she had a high fever.

Dermatomyositis

Dermatomyositis (DM) is an autoimmune, inflammatory disease of skin and skeletal muscle. It can occur at any age and carries an association with internal malignancy. The relative risk for malignancy in DM is up to 26.0. Women have a specific susceptibility for ovarian carcinoma. The skin signs of DM commonly precede myositis and are often the presenting feature of this serious, systemic illness.

CLINICAL FEATURES
Periorbital oedema and violaceous erythema of the eyelids is characteristic (the so-called 'heliotrope' rash) (**134**). Macular erythema often occurs elsewhere on the face as well the neck, upper back (the shawl sign), and upper chest (**135**). Scalp erythema is common. Gottron's papules are flat-topped, red lesions on the knuckles (distal and proximal interphalangeal joints) (**136**). Gottron's lines can be seen on the extensor surface of the fingers and backs of hands. Periungual erythema, prominent nail fold capillaries, and ragged cuticles are usually present but are not specific to DM. Red or violaceous plaques occur on the extensor surfaces of limbs. Very active skin involvement in DM can result in blistering and erosions. Muscle involvement usually presents as a symmetrical myositis with proximal limb weakness. Bulbar muscle weakness causes problems with speech and swallowing while diaphragmatic involvement leads to dyspnoea.

DIFFERENTIAL DIAGNOSIS
- Rosacea (papules, pustules, telangiectasiae, and erythema on the face).
- Seborrhoeic dermatitis (p. 20, erythema and scaling of the face, scalp, and chest).
- Systemic lupus erythematosus (p. 108, butterfly rash, periungual erythema, and systemic features).
- Subacute cutaneous lupus erythematosus (p. 110, annular and polycyclic eruption on upper torso).
- Mixed connective tissue disease (an overlap syndrome of systemic lupus erythematosus, systemic sclerosis, and myositis).
- Allergic contact dermatitis (p. 18, eczema in a localized area or unusual distribution).
- Phototoxic drug eruption (p. 222, eruption on exposed skin caused by a photosensitizing drug).

COMPLICATIONS
- Muscle involvement:
- – Proximal limb muscles: limb weakness.
- – Bulbar muscles: dysphagia/dysphonia.
- – Respiratory muscles: ventilatory dysfunction.
- Polyarthropathy.
- Vasculitis.
- Interstitial pneumonitis.
- Subcutaneous calcification.

INVESTIGATIONS
- Blood count, basic chemistry, liver function tests (as indicator of general health and as baseline for monitoring systemic therapy).
- ESR, CRP (inflammatory markers will be raised).
- ANA, complement, anti-dsDNA, -Sm, -Ro(SS-A), -La(SS-B), -RNP, -Jo-1, -Mi-2 antibodies, lupus anticoagulant, and anticardiolipin antibodies (ANA is positive in approximately 60%; anti-Jo-1 occurs more frequently in polymyositis and is associated with pneumonitis; anti-Mi-2 is specific but not sensitive for DM).
- Creatine phosphokinase (CPK), aldolase (CPK is the most reliable marker for active myositis).
- Muscle biopsy (may be negative since muscle inflammation can be patchy).
- Electromyography (EMG) (demonstrates typical myositis changes).
- Muscle magnetic resonance imaging (MRI) (may be more sensitive at identifying focal myositis).
- Skin biopsy for histopathology (lymphocytic infiltrate at the dermoepidermal junction with epidermal atrophy, basal vacuolar change, and apoptotic keratinocytes).
- The following should be performed if an underlying malignancy is suspected: chest radiography, abdomino-pelvic ultrasonography, cervical cytology, CT scan of neck, thorax, abdomen, and pelvis, mammography, upper and lower gastrointestinal endoscopy.

134 Dermatomyositis. In white skin the violaceous erythema of the eyelids is usually clearly visible (upper panel), whereas it is more difficult to appreciate in dark skin (lower panel). The inflammatory changes of the eyelids are accompanied by oedema.

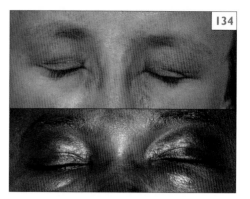

135 Dermatomyositis. This man with DM and associated bladder cancer presented with photosensitive erythema on exposed skin, including the V of the chest.

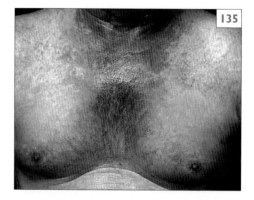

136 Dermatomyositis. There is periungual erythema, ragged cuticles, and dilated nail fold capillaries. The lesions on the fingers and knuckles are Gottron's papules.

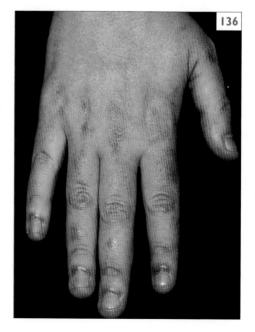

- Serum markers of malignancy: prostatic specific antigen (in men), carcinoembryonic antigen, alpha-fetoprotein, cancer antigen 125 (CA-125), carbohydrate antigen 19-9 (CA19-9).

IMMEDIATE MANAGEMENT
Topical therapy
- Corticosteroid ointment, twice per day (use for a restricted period):
     face: mildly potent.
     trunk and limbs: moderately potent or potent.

Systemic therapy
- Moderate- to high-dose oral corticosteroids (e.g. prednisolone 1 mg/kg/day), reducing with response.

Supportive therapy
- If acutely ill, admit to hospital for bed rest, investigations, and initiation of therapy.
- Patients with respiratory muscle involvement require daily spirometry assessment to monitor vital capacity.
- Patients with bulbar muscle involvement may require feeding via a nasogastric tube or gastrostomy.

LONG-TERM MANAGEMENT ISSUES
If appropriate, detailed investigations should be carried out to seek an underlying malignancy, particularly ovarian carcinoma in women. A steroid-sparing agent is often required, for example azathioprine 2–3 mg/kg/day, methotrexate 10–20 mg/week or mycophenolate mofetil 500–1500 mg twice per day. Pulsed intravenous methylprednisolone (500 mg or 1 g on 3 consecutive days) and/or intravenous immunoglobulin infusions (0.4 g/kg/day for 5 days) may also be effective to gain control of severe DM. In recalcitrant DM further long-term immunosuppressive therapy may be required with cyclophosphamide or ciclosporin. Prolonged use of systemic corticosteroids requires ongoing screening for diabetes and hypertension and prophylaxis against osteoporosis. Gastric protection with a proton pump inhibitor is often needed (e.g. omeprazole 20 mg once daily). Photoprotection with appropriate clothing, a hat, and a high protection factor topical sunscreen is advisable. Patients with DM often require management from a multidisciplinary team, including rheumatologists and dermatologists.

Bacterial diseases

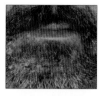 Impetigo

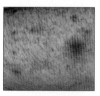 Folliculitis and furunculosis

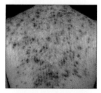 Hidradenitis suppurativa

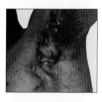 Acne conglobata and acne fulminans

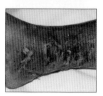 Erysipelas and cellulitis

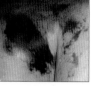 Necrotizing fasciitis

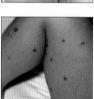 Septic vasculitis and infectious purpura fulminans

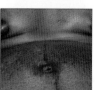 Lyme disease

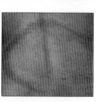 Toxic shock syndrome and staphylococcal scalded skin syndrome

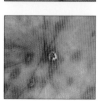 Syphilis

Impetigo

Impetigo is a superficial cutaneous infection caused by *Staphylococcus aureus* or rarely by group A streptococci. It is common in the young and especially where people live in close proximity with one another. Blistering, which can occur in impetigo, is caused by exfoliative toxins released by staphylococci. The rapid development of impetigo and its striking appearance often precipitate an acute presentation.

CLINICAL FEATURES

Impetigo commonly occurs on the face, often arising on the skin around the nose. Typically the initial lesion is a superficial blister which ruptures to leave an eroded area which may be sore or itchy. The erosion becomes covered by honey-coloured crust, indicative of *S. aureus* infection (**137**). In some cases of bullous impetigo (**138**) the blisters can be large and tense. Impetigo lesions have a surrounding red margin and tend to expand outwards. New lesions may arise close by the original crusted area.

DIFFERENTIAL DIAGNOSIS
- Herpes simplex virus infection (p. 142, grouped vesicles preceded by localized pain).
- Herpes zoster (p. 148, vesicles in a dermatomal distribution).
- Dermatophyte (tinea) infection (p. 154, annular lesion(s) with inflammatory margin).
- Allergic contact dermatitis (p. 18, eczema in a localized area or unusual distribution).
- Pemphigus foliaceous (p. 68, blisters and scaling).
- Bullous pemphigoid (p. 66, itchy erythema with large tense blisters).

COMPLICATIONS
- Regional lymphadenopathy.
- Erysipelas/cellulitis.

INVESTIGATIONS
- The diagnosis is usually made clinically.
- Skin swab from lesion for bacteriology.
- Skin swab from carrier sites (nose, axillae, perineum) for bacteriology.

IMMEDIATE MANAGEMENT
Topical therapy
- Remove the crusts with warm saline or a dilute solution of potassium permanganate.
- Topical antibiotic ointment (e.g. fusidic acid or mupiricin) to affected area three times per day for 7 days.

Systemic therapy
- In extensive involvement: oral antibiotics, e.g. flucloxacillin 500 mg four times per day for 7 days (erythromycin if penicillin-allergic).
- Antibiotics may need to be altered according to bacteriological sensitivities (e.g. in streptococcal or methicillin-resistant *Staphylococcus aureus* (MRSA) infections).

LONG-TERM MANAGEMENT ISSUES

In recurrent impetigo, the source of *S. aureus* should be sought and eradicated. As well as swabbing carrier sites (nose, axillae, perineum), close family and personal contacts may also need to be screened for carriage of *S. aureus*. Nasal carriage needs to be treated with fusidic acid or mupiricin ointment or chlorhexidine cream applied to the anterior nares three times per day for 7 days. For other positive carriage sites use chlorhexidine body-wash twice per day for 7 days. Following treatment, carrier sites need to be reswabbed to ensure eradication of *S. aureus*. In some parts of the world, MRSA is a particular problem and alternative antibiotics may be necessary.

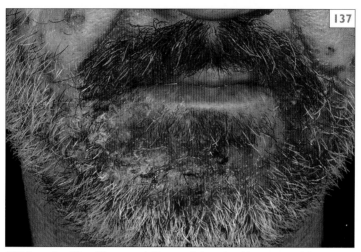

137 Impetigo. The skin around the mouth is red and has an overlying golden crust, which is typical in impetigo.

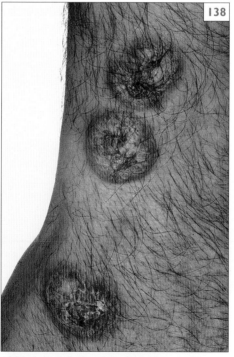

138 Impetigo. Bullous impetigo on the wrist. Flaccid blisters without crusting.

Folliculitis and furunculosis

Folliculitis is a pustular inflammation of hair follicles. A furuncle is an abscess that evolves from a folliculitis lesion. *S. aureus* is the most common infecting organism in both conditions. Gram-negative folliculitis occurs in a number of unusual clinical situations, such as bathing in water colonized by *Pseudomonas* spp. which can occur in ponds, lakes, and hot tubs. Occlusion of the skin predisposes to folliculitis, such as on the back of a recumbent patient, or following the frequent application of a greasy emollient.

CLINICAL FEATURES
In folliculitis, red papules or pustules, centred on hair follicles, develop within hair-bearing skin (**139–141**). Individual lesions may be painful. The limbs, especially legs, are commonly affected in staphylococcal folliculitis, the torso is typically involved in Gram-negative folliculitis. Folliculitis decalvans is a form of staphylococcal scalp infection causing irreversible scarring alopecia. *Pityrosporum* folliculitis is a yeast infection occurring on the back. A furuncle is a tender, warm, red nodule which becomes fluctuant, eventually pointing before breaking down and discharging pus (**142**). The back of the neck is the most common site for a furuncle.

DIFFERENTIAL DIAGNOSIS
- Acne vulgaris (p. 124, comedones, papules, pustules, and nodules on face and torso).
- Candidiasis (p. 158, nonfollicular, superficial pustules especially in flexures).
- Hidradenitis suppurativa (p. 122, abscesses, nodules, sinuses, and scarring especially in flexures).
- Pseudofolliculitis barbae (an irritant perifolliculitis caused by in-growing beard hairs).
- Pruritic papular eruption (widespread itchy papules occurring in HIV infection).

COMPLICATIONS
- Regional lymphadenopathy.
- Fever and malaise (in extensive furunculosis).

INVESTIGATIONS
- The diagnosis is usually made clinically.
- Skin swab from lesion for bacteriology.
- Skin swab from carrier sites (nose, axillae, perineum) for bacteriology.

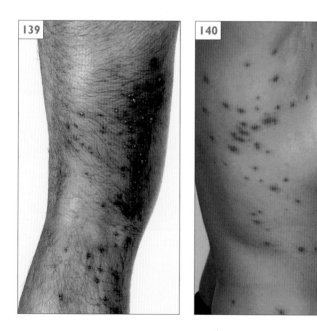

139 Folliculitis. There are numerous pustules centred on hair follicles surrounded by a zone of erythema.

140 Gram-negative folliculitis. Multiple folliculitis lesions occurring after bathing in water colonized by *Pseudomonas aeruginosa*.

141 Folliculitis. In some cases of folliculitis the pustules are only seen on close inspection.

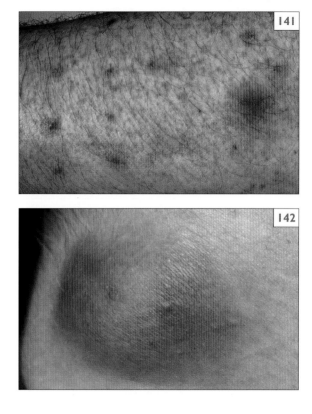

142 Furunculosis. A solitary red, tender furuncle, which has yet to point.

IMMEDIATE MANAGEMENT
Topical therapy
- Topical mupiricin or fusidic acid ointment or clindamycin gel applied to the affected areas twice per day for 7 days.
- Furuncles require incision and drainage if the lesions do not discharge spontaneously.

Systemic therapy
- Flucloxacillin 500 mg four times per day for 7 days (erythromycin if penicillin-allergic).
- Antibiotics may need to be altered according to bacteriological sensitivities (e.g. in MRSA infections).
- For Gram-negative folliculitis use ciprofloxacin 500 mg twice per day for 7 days (altered according to bacteriological sensitivities).

LONG-TERM MANAGEMENT ISSUES
In recurrent staphylococcal folliculitis and furunculosis, a source of *S. aureus* should be sought and eradicated. As well as swabbing carrier sites (nose, axillae, perineum), close family and personal contacts may also need to be screened for carriage of *S. aureus*. Nasal carriage needs to be treated with fusidic acid or mupiricin ointment or chlorhexidine cream applied to the anterior nares three times per day for 7 days. For other positive carriage sites use chlorhexidine body-wash twice per day for 7 days. Following treatment, carrier sites need to be reswabbed to ensure eradication of *S. aureus*.

Hidradenitis suppurativa

Hidradenitis suppurativa (HS) is a dermatosis in which inflammation of the apocrine sweat glands produces nodules, abscesses, discharging sinuses, and scarring. It occurs slightly more commonly in women who often report premenstrual and menstrual flares. Despite the involvement of suppurative inflammation the role of bacteria in the aetiology of HS is unknown. HS generally runs a chronic course, however acute exacerbations often cause the patient to seek an urgent opinion.

CLINICAL FEATURES

HS occurs on the skin of the axillae, groins, breasts, buttocks, and anogenital area, which are the sites of apocrine glands. The earliest lesion is an acutely inflamed nodule ('blind boil') which is painful and tender. Deep extension leads to induration of surrounding skin with thick, tethering bands of scarring. After a few weeks pus and blood may discharge from the nodular lesion, giving rise to a chronically leaking sinus (**143, 144**). Comedones (often bridged or with multiple openings) are a feature of HS and help to distinguish it from bacterial furunculosis. Extensive involvement of the axillae and anogenital skin is uncomfortable and may cause functional and mobility problems.

DIFFERENTIAL DIAGNOSIS

- Bacterial folliculitis and furunculosis (p. 120, follicular pustules or abscesses often on the limbs or neck).
- Acne conglobata (p. 124, nodules, pustules, comedones on face and torso).
- Crohn's disease (inflammation at the perineum with sinuses and fistulae).
- Lymphogranuloma venereum (inguinal lymphadenopathy with sinuses).

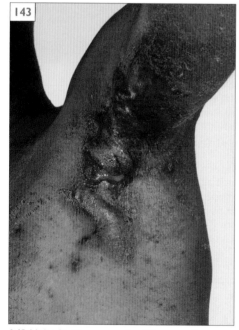

143 Hidradenitis suppurativa. There are large abscesses and thick bands of scarring in the axilla. A sinus is leaking pus.

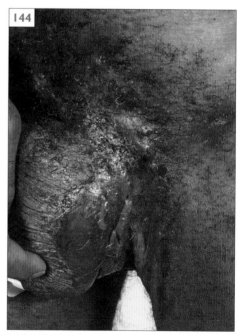

144 Hidradenitis suppurativa. The groin is a typical site of involvement. In this case there are inflamed nodules and a sinus producing pus.

COMPLICATIONS

- Arthralgia (with extensive HS).
- Anaemia (of chronic inflammation).
- Hypoalbuminaemia (with longstanding inflammation and sinus discharge).
- Deep extension into pelvic organs.
- Squamous cell carcinoma (in longstanding cases).
- Depression.

INVESTIGATIONS

- The diagnosis is usually made clinically.
- Skin swabs for bacteriology (often negative, however pathogenic bacteria must be sought and treated; organisms often found in HS include *S. aureus*, *Streptococcus milleri*, and anaerobic streptococci).

In severe involvement:
- Blood count (a normochromic, normocytic anaemia and leucocytosis may occur).
- Basic chemistry, liver function tests (as indicators of general health and systemic complications).
- ESR, CRP (inflammatory markers are raised in active, extensive HS).

IMMEDIATE MANAGEMENT
Topical therapy

- Surgical incision and drainage of a tender abscess is sometimes necessary.
- Potassium permanganate soaks to cleanse discharging areas.
- Intralesional triamcinolone injection (only if bacterial infection has been excluded).

Systemic therapy

- Systemic antibiotics to treat confirmed bacterial infection.
- Adequate analgesia.
- Erythromycin 500 mg four times per day given for 2 weeks is often helpful when waiting for bacteriological results. It can also be useful if the swabs are negative.
- A 10-week course of rifampicin 300 mg twice per day and clindamycin 150–300 mg twice per day may settle acute exacerbations.
- For severe, acute exacerbations consider prednisolone 20–30 mg/day, reducing with response (only if bacterial infection has been excluded).

LONG-TERM MANAGEMENT ISSUES

Careful hygiene to affected areas is important, as is loss of weight in the obese. Topical antibiotics, such as clindamycin, may be helpful in controlling exacerbations. Oral antibiotics given for up to 6 months (e.g. erythromycin 500 mg twice per day, minocycline 100 mg once daily, or clindamycin 150 mg twice per day) can settle HS in many cases. In women the oral contraceptive pill can control HS, particularly those with a high oestrogen/progestogen ratio or those containing cyproterone acetate. Systemic retinoids, isotretinoin and acitretin, may induce a remission in some cases. Infliximab infusions have been used successfully in extensive, active HS. Established scars and sinuses can be excised while large areas of involved skin are sometimes excised and grafted.

Acne conglobata and acne fulminans

Both acne conglobata (AC) and acne fulminans (AF) are rare, aggressive forms of acne vulgaris. The severe systemic inflammation in AF is caused by sensitivity to *Propionibacterium acnes*, however in AC, and in other forms of acne, this bacterium is only one of a number of pathogenetic triggers. The extensive inflammation in both types, and the constitutional symptoms in AF, necessitate prompt therapeutic intervention.

CLINICAL FEATURES
AC and AF occur predominantly in teenage boys. The onset is characterized by a rapid development of numerous painful, large, inflammatory pustules and nodules (**145, 146**). Some lesions become purpuric, others haemorrhagic. Large nodules can fuse to form draining sinuses, other lesions become eroded or ulcerated. There are also numerous comedones (blackheads) which can be grouped. In both forms the back, shoulders, and chest are predominantly involved as well as the face. AF is accompanied by an acute systemic upset with multiple manifestations (see below).

DIFFERENTIAL DIAGNOSIS
- Hidradenitis suppurativa (p. 122, abscesses, nodules, sinuses, and scarring especially in flexures).
- Bacterial folliculitis and furunculosis (p. 120, follicular pustules or abscesses often on the limbs or neck).

COMPLICATIONS
In acne fulminans:
- Fever and malaise.
- Myalgia, arthralgia, and arthritis.
- Hepatosplenomegaly (splenomegaly may be painful).
- Bone pain (from aseptic osteolytic bone lesions).
- Erythema nodosum.

INVESTIGATIONS
The diagnosis is usually made clinically.
In acne fulminans the following should be performed:
- Blood count (normochromic, normocytic anaemia, and leucocytosis may occur).
- Basic chemistry, liver function tests (alkaline phosphatase may be elevated).
- ESR, CRP (inflammatory markers are raised).
- Urinalysis (may show microscopic haematuria and proteinuria).
- Skin swabs for bacteriology (to exclude secondary infection).
- Blood cultures (to exclude systemic sepsis).
- Skeletal radiographs or radioisotope bone scans (may show osteolytic bone lesions corresponding to sites of bone pain).

IMMEDIATE MANAGEMENT
Topical therapy
- Potassium permanganate soaks once daily to cleanse discharging areas.
- Corticosteroid ointment, twice per day: trunk and limbs: potent or superpotent.

Systemic therapy
- Isotretinoin (0.5–1 mg/kg orally for 3–5 months) AND
- Tapering course of prednisolone (0.5 mg/kg daily and reduce by 5 mg each week).
- Systemic antibiotics may be required if secondary infection occurs.

Supportive therapy
- In acne fulminans the patient may need to be admitted to hospital for bed rest and initiation of therapy.

LONG-TERM MANAGEMENT ISSUES
AF generally resolves after several months and does not recur. AC can persist for many years, despite active treatment. Lesions heal slowly with extensive scarring.

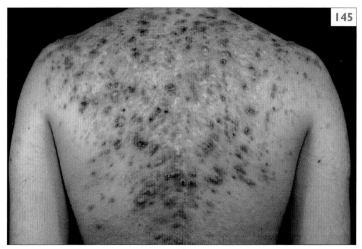

145 Acne fulminans. There are numerous inflamed nodules some with necrotic centres on this young man's back. The skin signs are accompanied by systemic features, such as fever and arthralgia.

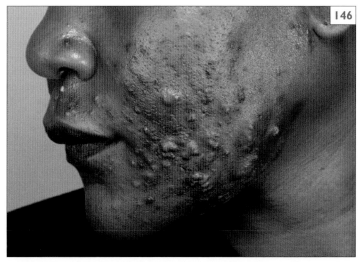

146 Acne conglobata. Large inflammatory nodules on the cheek and a cyst on the jawline.

Erysipelas and cellulitis

Erysipelas and cellulitis are acute infections of the dermis and subcutis, caused by group A or other streptococci. *S. aureus* and other bacteria are causative in a minority of cases. In erysipelas there is infection of the dermis and superficial subcutaneous tissues, whereas in cellulitis the infection extends deeper into the subcutis. Pathogenic bacteria enter the skin through an abrasion or via a breach in the skin produced by another dermatosis, e.g. tinea pedis. Cellulitis is a common complication of lymphoedema. Erysipelas and cellulitis are serious infections accompanied by a severe, systemic illness and significant morbidity.

CLINICAL FEATURES

Erysipelas and cellulitis both present acutely with a hot, painful, red, oedematous area of skin. Erysipelas most commonly occurs on the face and is usually unilateral (**147**). Cellulitis typically occurs as an ascending inflammation of the leg or can complicate a wound or ulcer (**148–150**). Since the infection is superficial in erysipelas the margins are more clearly demarcated than in cellulitis. In cellulitis blisters and ulceration may develop within the area of involvement (**149, 151**). Pain from regional lymphadenopathy and fever may precede the appearance of cutaneous signs. Haemorrhagic cellulitis is a hyperacute form in which purpura occurs within the zone of oedematous erythema (**151**).

DIFFERENTIAL DIAGNOSIS
Cellulitis of the leg
- Deep venous thrombosis (limb swelling, erythema, and pain).
- Necrotizing fasciitis (p. 128, spreading zone of painful erythema with swelling and purpura).
- Venous eczema (p. 16, eczema on the lower leg, usually with other signs of venous incompetence).
- Allergic contact dermatitis (p. 18, eczema in a localized area or unusual distribution).
- Dependency syndrome (p. 96, bilateral swollen, red legs).

Erysipelas of the face
- Rosacea (erythema on the face with papules, pustules, and telangiectasiae).
- Allergic contact dermatitis (p. 18, eczema in a localized area or unusual distribution).
- Lupus erythematosus (p. 106, circumscribed red plaques and patches, scarring in discoid lupus erythematosus).
- Dermatomyositis (p. 114, violaceous eyelid erythema and oedema, Gottron's papules, and myositis).

COMPLICATIONS
- Fever and rigors.
- Lymphangitis and lymphadenopathy.
- Vomiting.
- Nephritis (following infection with the nephritogenic strain of *Streptococcus*).
- Septicaemic shock.

INVESTIGATIONS
- The diagnosis is usually made clinically.
- Skin swabs for bacteriology (culture of a skin swab produces a positive result in only 25% of cases).
- Blood cultures (a blood culture produces a positive result in only 25% of cases).
- Streptococcal serology (a positive ASOT can be useful to confirm streptococcal infection).
- Blood count (neutrophilia is likely).
- Basic chemistry, liver function tests (as indicators of systemic complications and general health).
- ESR, CRP (raised CRP).

IMMEDIATE MANAGEMENT
Topical therapy
- Blisters should be decompressed and a nonadhesive, absorbant dressing applied over any exudative or ulcerated areas.
- In limb cellulitis an elasticated tubular bandage or gentle compression bandaging can help to reduce oedema.

147 Erysipelas. There is an extensive zone of well demarcated erythema and oedema involving the left cheek, nose, and forehead. The patient was febrile and had cervical lymphadenopathy.

148 Cellulitis. There is erythema and swelling of the left lower leg and ankle. The patient had a high fever.

149 Cellulitis. Swelling, erythema, and petechiae of the leg. At the ankle there is ulceration with infected slough.

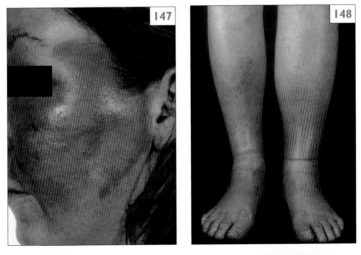

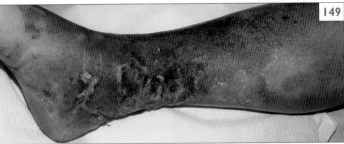

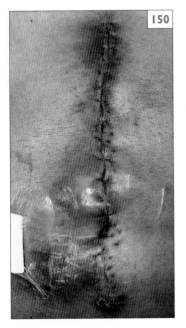

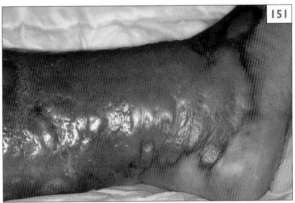

151 Cellulitis. Bullous and haemorrhagic cellulitis. Severe skin sepsis was associated with acute renal failure in this patient.

150 Cellulitis. Erythema spreading from a recent surgical wound.

Systemic therapy

- Mild involvement: oral phenoxymethylpenicillin 500 mg + flucloxacillin 500 mg, both four times per day for 7 days.
- Moderate and severe involvement: IV benzylpenicillin 1.2 g + IV flucloxacillin 1–2 g, both four times per day for 5–7 days.
- Use IV erythromycin 50 mg/kg/day in four divided doses or clarithromycin 500 mg twice daily if allergic to penicillin.
- Use IV vancomycin 1 g once daily in patients known to be infected by MRSA.
- Bites from cats and dogs (and humans) can give rise to cellulitis caused by oral aerobes and anaerobes: in these cases antibiotics given should include broad-spectrum anaerobic cover.
- In haemorrhagic cellulitis oral corticosteroids (e.g. prednisolone 0.5 mg/kg daily) may be required to control the inflammation.

Supportive therapy

- With moderate and severe involvement admit to hospital for bed rest, monitoring of vital signs, and intravenous therapy.
- Elevate affected area.

LONG-TERM MANAGEMENT ISSUES

If a portal of bacterial entry is present, i.e. tinea pedis, then this should be treated appropriately. Recurrent erysipelas or cellulitis will damage the lymphatics and may lead to lymphoedema. In these patients long-term low-dose antibiotics (e.g. penicillin V 500 mg once daily) and active management of the lymphoedema may be helpful at preventing recurrent episodes of cellulitis.

Necrotizing fasciitis

Necrotizing fasciitis (NF) is a life-threatening infection of deep dermis, subcutis, and muscle. Since the infection spreads along deep fascial planes the overlying skin is initially intact until secondary gangrene occurs. NF may follow surgery or minor trauma and is more likely to occur in immunosuppressed patients (including diabetics, alcoholics, and patients with malignancy). Other insults associated with NF include penetrating injuries, intravenous drug use, and burns. Type I NF is caused by mixed aerobes and anaerobes, type II NF is caused by group A streptococci and occasionally staphylococci. NF usually runs a rapidly progressive course and therefore early recognition and intervention are necessary to reduce mortality.

CLINICAL FEATURES

Initially there is an area of pain and swelling with overlying poorly defined erythema. Often the condition affects a limb or the extremities; involvement of genitalia is known as Fournier's gangrene. An early clue to the diagnosis is severe, localized pain which is out of proportion to the clinical signs on the skin. The area of erythema and oedema extends swiftly over the next 24–72 hr and produces purpura, blistering, and skin necrosis (152, 153). If untreated, NF usually results in a rapid clinical deterioration. In fulminant cases the patient may die within 24 hr of symptom onset.

DIFFERENTIAL DIAGNOSIS

- Haemorrhagic cellulitis (p. 126, zone of spreading erythema with purpura; fever).
- Pyoderma gangrenosum (p. 92, a painful, destructive ulcer with dusky margins).
- Widespread cutaneous necrosis (p. 88, large areas of purpura with a variety of causes).

COMPLICATIONS

- Fever.
- Streptococcal toxic shock syndrome.
- DIC.
- Cardiovascular collapse.
- Renal failure.
- Adult respiratory distress syndrome.
- Multiorgan failure.

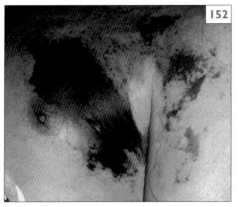

152 Necrotizing fasciitis. There is a large ecchymotic patch on the chest. Purpuric areas, indicating underlying necrosis, have also spread on to the adjacent shoulder and upper arm.

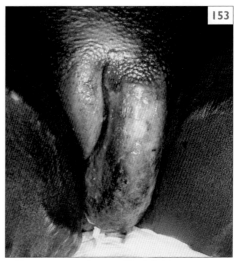

153 Necrotizing fasciitis. The left labium majora is grossly swollen, dusky, and incipiently necrotic.

INVESTIGATIONS
- The diagnosis is usually made clinically.
- Blood count (neutrophilia).
- Basic chemistry, liver function tests (renal impairment with hyperkalaemia occurs early).
- Clotting studies (DIC may occur).
- ESR, CRP (greatly raised).
- CPK, LDH (will be raised with muscle involvement).
- Blood cultures, streptococcal serology.
- Skin swab and aspirate of blister fluid for bacteriology.
- Plain radiographs (gas can be detected in subcutaneous fascial planes).
- MRI scan (T1 MRI imaging can identify deep tissue necrosis and may assist the planning of surgery).
- Deep incisional skin biopsy for histopathology (early lesions: deep dermal and pannicular oedema and haemorrhage; advanced lesions: necrosis at all levels, including myonecrosis, intravascular thrombosis, neutrophil infiltrate, Gram-positive cocci).

IMMEDIATE MANAGEMENT
Local therapy
- Early, aggressive surgical debridement is the mainstay of effective treatment.

Systemic therapy
- If type I NF is suspected, administer broad-spectrum antibiotics to cover aerobes and anaerobes.
- For type II NF, intravenous infusion of clindamycin 1.2 g four times per day.
- Addition of further antibiotics should be guided by expert microbiological advice.

Supportive therapy
- Admit to intensive care unit (ICU) or high-dependency unit (HDU) for close monitoring and cardiovascular, respiratory, and metabolic support.
- Opiate analgesia is often necessary.

LONG-TERM MANAGEMENT ISSUES
If the patient survives then plastic surgical reconstruction is usually required to resurface the surgically debrided area.

Septic vasculitis and infectious purpura fulminans

Vasculitis with cutaneous involvement can complicate septicaemia. Septic vasculitis is most commonly associated with meningococcal infection (*Neisseria meningitidis*) but can also be caused by *Streptococcus*, *Staphylococcus*, *Gonococcus*, and *Pseudomonas*. Meningococcaemia may also precipitate purpura fulminans, a skin necrosis syndrome caused by dermal vascular thrombosis in the setting of DIC. Vascular thrombosis follows infection-induced clotting factor activation, platelet consumption, and fibrin formation. Other infections can also trigger DIC, including *Streptococcus*, *Staphylococcus*, *Haemophilus*, and varicella zoster virus. Septic vasculitis and infectious purpura fulminans are medical emergencies necessitating early diagnosis, immediate antibiotic treatment, and intensive supportive care to prevent a fatal outcome.

CLINICAL FEATURES

The patient is usually extremely ill. Early infection may be associated with a nonspecific maculopapular exanthem, however purpura tends to develop 6–12 hr into the illness. The purpuric lesions may be small and few in number, or numerous and scattered widely over the trunk and limbs (**154**). *Pseudomonas* infections are typified by haemorrhagic lesions which are solitary or few in number and known as eccthyma gangrenosum (**155**). In full-blown purpura fulminans there are large zones of skin necrosis, particularly in dependent areas, which often display retiform (branching) or stellate patterns (**156**). Ischaemia of acral tissues, known as symmetrical peripheral gangrene, commonly accompanies infectious purpura fulminans (**157**).

DIFFERENTIAL DIAGNOSIS
- Cutaneous small vessel vasculitis (p. 82, palpable purpura on lower legs).
- Thrombocytopenic petechiae (pinpoint macular purpura).
- Cutaneous emboli (p. 86, purpuric lesions on acral skin with livedo reticularis).
- Thrombophilia disorders (large stellate purpuric patches).

- Widespread cutaneous necrosis (p. 88, large areas of purpura with a variety of causes).
- Rocky Mountain spotted fever (p. 177, extensive petechial or purpuric eruption following tick bite).

COMPLICATIONS
- Fever and malaise.
- Myalgia.
- Abdominal pain.
- Septicaemic shock.
- DIC.
- Cardiovascular collapse.
- Renal failure.
- Adult respiratory distress syndrome.
- Multiorgan failure.
- With infection by *Neisseria meningitidis*:
- Meningitis (headache, photophobia, vomiting, neck stiffness).
- Signs of raised intracranial pressure.

INVESTIGATIONS
- Blood count, basic chemistry, liver function tests (initially neutrophilia, later leucopenia, severe thrombocytopenia; renal impairment).
- ESR, CRP (greatly raised).
- Clotting studies: PT, APTT, TT, FDPs, D-dimers (DIC produces prolonged PT, APTT, and TT, reduced fibrinogen level, high level of FDPs and D-dimers).
- Blood culture (*Neisseria meningitidis*; septicaemia with other organisms can also produce purpura).
- Brain imaging: CT or MRI (prior to lumbar puncture if raised intracranial pressure suspected).
- Cerebrospinal fluid (CSF) microscopy and culture (in meningococcal meningitis, direct microscopy shows diplococci, culture will grow *Neisseria meningitidis*).
- Skin scrapings for microscopy (direct microscopy shows diplococci).
- Skin biopsy for histopathology (microvascular damage with fibrinoid changes, a neutrophil infiltrate, occlusive thrombi, and red cell extravasation; Gram-negative diplococci in endothelial cells and neutrophils in meningococcal septicaemia).

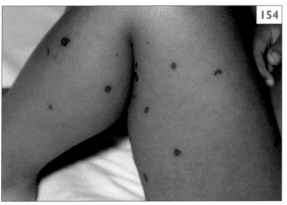

154 Septic vasculitis. There are several small necrotic lesions in this patient with meningococcal meningitis.

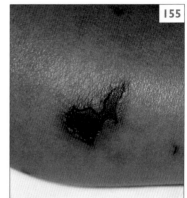

155 Eccthyma gangrenosum. An area of skin necrosis with straight, irregular margins which was associated with *Pseudomonas* septicaemia.

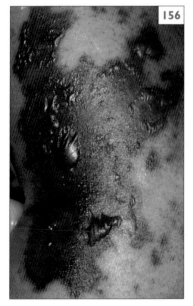

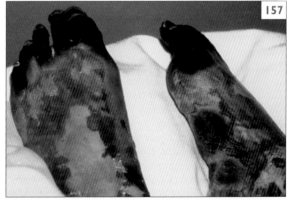

157 Infectious purpura fulminans. Symmetrical peripheral gangrene of the toes in a patient with meningococcal purpura fulminans.

156 Infectious purpura fulminans. A large area of blistering skin necrosis with a stellate outline in a patient with meningococcal septicaemia.

IMMEDIATE MANAGEMENT
Systemic therapy

- If meningococcal septicaemia is suspected, administer intravenous antibiotics immediately. Since other organisms can cause a purpuric eruption similar to meningococcal infection (e.g. *Streptococcus pneumoniae* and *Haemophilus influenzae* type B) a third-generation cephalosporin is the appropriate choice of antibiotic until cultures are available, e.g. IV cefotaxime 1 g twice per day, or ceftriaxone 1 g once daily.
- If it is known that the patient has acute meningococcaemia give IV benzylpenicillin 2.4 g every 4 hr.
- In infectious purpura fulminans consider infusion of recombinant human activated protein C.

Supportive therapy

- Admit to ICU for close monitoring of cardiovascular, respiratory, and renal function.

LONG-TERM MANAGEMENT ISSUES

Peripheral gangrene requires either debridement of necrotic tissue or amputation. All close contacts to a patient with acute meningococcaemia should receive prophylactic rifampicin: adults – 600 mg twice daily for 2 days; children – 10 mg/kg twice daily for 2 days; children under 1 year – 5 mg/kg twice daily for 2 days. In some countries there is a meningococcal vaccine available which protects against serogroups A, C, Y, and W-135; it is given to young adults congregated in large groups, e.g. university students, military recruits. Chronic meningococcaemia is a rare disease characterized by recurrent episodes of fever, arthralgias, and an eruption consisting of red macules, papules, and plaques which develop 12–24 hr after the onset of the fever. The skin lesions develop into tender nodules before resolving.

Lyme disease

Lyme disease is a multisystem disorder caused by infection with the spirochaete *Borrelia burgdorferi*. *Ixodes* ticks are the primary vectors for Lyme borreliosis and the disease occurs where the tick is endemic. The most common secondary vectors are sheep and deer. It is important to diagnose Lyme disease in the early stages so that appropriate treatment can halt progression to serious, systemic involvement.

CLINICAL FEATURES

Three to 30 days following the tick bite the papular reaction develops into an annular lesion, called erythema chronicum migrans (ECM), which slowly expands outwards over several weeks (**158**). With time the centre of the lesion clears but the margin can reach many centimetres in diameter (**159**). Untreated ECM generally disappears spontaneously after several weeks. ECM may appear at any site but the legs are most commonly affected. Lesions may be solitary or multiple.

DIFFERENTIAL DIAGNOSIS

- Insect bite reaction (p. 164, itchy, urticated nodule with central punctum).
- Dermatophyte (tinea) infection (p. 154, annular lesion with inflammatory margin).
- Fixed drug eruption (p. 228, deep red circular patch, sometimes blisters).
- Annular erythema (ring-shaped red lesions).
- Granuloma annulare (red–brown circular patch often on acral skin).
- Morphoea (localized patch of scleroderma).

COMPLICATIONS

If untreated, Lyme disease can result in:
- Neurological disease: meningitis, encephalomyelitis, cranial nerve palsies.
- Rheumatological disease: arthritis.
- Cardiological disease: carditis, atrioventricular block.

INVESTIGATIONS

- Serum for *B. burgdorferi* serology (may be negative in the first few weeks post-inoculation but with time will become positive).
- Skin biopsy for histopathology (superficial and deep perivascular and interstitial lymphohistiocytic infiltrate containing plasma cells; Warthin–Starry stain can identify spirochaetes).

IMMEDIATE MANAGEMENT
Systemic therapy
If erythema chronicum migrans is suspected treat with oral antibiotics:
- Amoxicillin 500–1000 mg three times per day for 3 weeks or doxycycline 100 mg twice per day for 3 weeks.

LONG-TERM MANAGEMENT ISSUES
Disseminated Lyme disease should be treated with IV ceftriaxone 2 g daily for 2 weeks or IV benzylpenicillin 2.4 g daily for 2 weeks. Consider prophylactic treatment after tick bite in endemic areas.

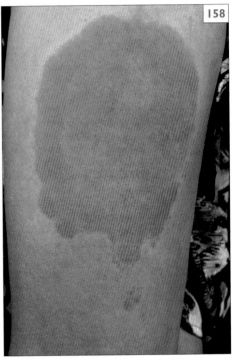

158 Lyme disease. Erythema chronicum migrans is a nonscaly discoid or annular lesion which expands outwards from the tick bite over several weeks.

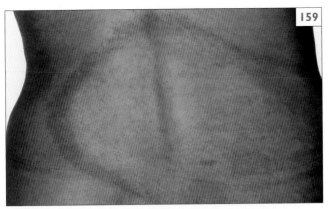

159 Lyme disease. The annular lesion of erythema chronicum migrans can reach many centimetres in diameter.

Toxic shock syndrome and staphylococcal scalded skin syndrome

Toxic shock syndrome (TSS) and staphylococcal scalded skin syndrome (SSSS) are both toxin-mediated illnesses caused by a toxin-producing *S. aureus*. In TSS the causative strains of *S. aureus* produce toxic shock syndrome toxin-1 (TSST-1). TSS was initially most commonly seen in young women following colonization by *S. aureus* of high-absorbancy tampons. Nowadays nonmenstrual TSS is more usual and can occur following staphylococcal infection of burns, wounds, intrauterine contraceptive devices, and in postpartum infections. TSS can also be caused by group A *Streptococcus*. SSSS is usually seen in young children, however it can uncommonly occur in adults, especially those with renal failure. SSSS is caused by phage group II strains of *S. aureus* which produce exfoliative toxins. Toxin-mediated skin cleavage in SSSS occurs at a high level within the epidermis and therefore involved skin does not become fully denuded.

CLINICAL FEATURES
Toxic shock syndrome
Patients are usually extremely ill with a high fever, headache, myalgia, vomiting, and diarrhoea. There is a widespread macular or scarlatiniform erythema which starts on the torso and spreads centrifugally (**160**). Oedema of the face and hands is often marked and there is an intense erythema of the buccal, pharyngeal, and conjunctival mucosae. Occasionally vesicles and bullae may occur. Purpuric areas may develop if there is significant thrombocytopenia (**161**). Examination must include a vaginal inspection for any retained tampons or other material. Desquamation of the hands and feet occurs 2 weeks after the acute illness.

Staphylococcal scalded skin syndrome
Painful erythema occurs initially in the flexures or on the face. Within a few hours the erythema becomes generalized. Thereafter flaccid blisters develop at pressure points and sites of skin shearing. Nikolsky's sign is positive. The blisters rupture easily leaving moist, red, tender skin. Involvement of the face produces crusting and oedema. Widespread desquamation occurs over the next 3–5 days.

DIFFERENTIAL DIAGNOSIS
Toxic shock syndrome
• SSSS (painful, superficial skin peeling on areas of erythema).
• Viral exanthem (p. 140, widespread morbilliform exanthem with flu-like symptoms).
• Stevens–Johnson syndrome/toxic epidermal necrolysis (p. 230, mucocutaneous blistering with large areas of epidermal loss).
• Rocky Mountain spotted fever (p. 177, extensive petechial or purpuric eruption following tick bite).

Staphylococcal scalded skin syndrome
• Bullous impetigo (p. 118, erythema, tense blisters, and honey-coloured crust).
• Pemphigus vulgaris (p. 68, vesicles, bullae, and erosions, usually involves the mouth).
• TSS (generalized scarlatiniform erythema, oedema of the face and hands, and erythema of the mucosae).
• Stevens–Johnson syndrome/toxic epidermal necrolysis (p. 230, mucocutaneous blistering with large areas of epidermal loss).

COMPLICATIONS
• Fever, headache, and confusion.
• Hypotension.
• Myalgia.
• Gastrointestinal upset.
• Renal failure.
• Adult respiratory distress syndrome.
• Circulatory shock.

INVESTIGATIONS

- Blood count (leucocytosis, low platelets in TSS).
- Basic chemistry (renal impairment/failure in TSS).
- Liver function tests (raised transaminases in TSS).
- Clotting studies (INR, APTT may be prolonged).
- CRP (elevated).
- High vaginal swab or skin swab for microbiology (in menstrual TSS a smear from a vaginal swab will reveal clusters of Gram-positive cocci; culture will yield TSST-1-producing *S. aureus*. In SSSS swab of blister is negative; *S. aureus* is cultured from nose, pharynx, or pyogenic focus).
- Blood culture.
- Skin biopsy for histopathology (TSS: confluent epidermal necrolysis, vacuolar alteration of the dermoepidermal junction, subepidermal splitting with a minimal inflammatory dermal infiltrate; SSSS: epidermal cleavage at the granular layer, no inflammatory cells, no organisms).

IMMEDIATE MANAGEMENT

Local therapy

- General emollient therapy.
- In TSS remove source of infection and clean infected sites.

Systemic therapy

- Intravenous antibiotics are needed: first line, in both TSS and SSSS, is flucloxacillin 500 mg four times per day for 7 days.

Supportive therapy

- Admit to HDU for close monitoring of cardiovascular, respiratory, and renal function.

LONG-TERM MANAGEMENT ISSUES

TSS is associated with serious systemic morbidity and a significant mortality, however if the correct treatment is administered early then most patients recover. Some patients have a period of prolonged fatigue after TSS. Telogen effluvium and Beau's lines are also commonly seen post-TSS. SSSS in adults is associated with a much worse prognosis than in children and is accompanied by a considerable mortality.

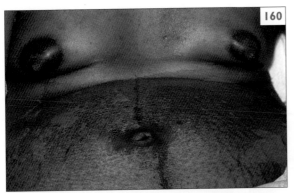

160 Toxic shock syndrome. Desquamation occurring 10 days after an acute toxic erythema. In this patient TSS was triggered by a postpartum vaginal infection with *S. aureus*.

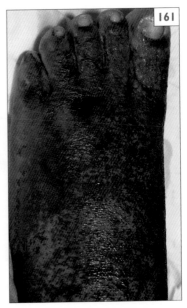

161 Toxic shock syndrome. Same patient as in **160**. Purpura and blistering occurred on the hands and feet. TSS can cause thrombocytopenia and a coagulopathy.

Syphilis

Syphilis is caused by the spirochaete *Treponema pallidum*. In the early stages the disease is highly infectious and is spread principally by sexual intercourse. The initial signs of primary and secondary syphilis are found on the skin and mucous membranes. Primary syphilis is characterized by a chancre which develops 2–6 weeks after infection. Following haematogenous and lymphatic spread of treponemes the secondary stage of syphilis appears 3–6 weeks after the chancre. Secondary syphilis is often characterized by a rash which, along with systemic symptoms, usually causes the patient to seek an urgent opinion.

CLINICAL FEATURES
Primary syphilis
The chancre starts as a papule usually on the genital skin but can occur on the anus, lips, or within the oral cavity. In men it commonly occurs on the glans penis (**162**) or on the underside of the prepuce. In women it often develops on the labia, commonly at the posterior commissure, however the chancre may be on the cervix and therefore easily missed. It develops into a painless, indurated, well demarcated ulcer approximately 1 cm in diameter. The chancre heals spontaneously within a few weeks but is still present in 25% of patients with secondary syphilis.

Secondary syphilis
Secondary syphilis is characterized by a red, nonitchy rash. The eruption is composed of numerous circular or oval lesions, initially macular but becoming papular with time, measuring 0.5–2 cm in diameter and usually widely and symmetrically disseminated on the face, trunk, and limbs (**163**). Circular, pink lesions, which may be scaly, are commonly seen on palmo-plantar skin (**164, 165**). Secondary syphilis can also involve the scalp resulting in patchy alopecia, producing a 'moth-eaten' appearance. Mucous membrane lesions in secondary syphilis are characterized by coalescent grey patches and shallow oval ulcers,

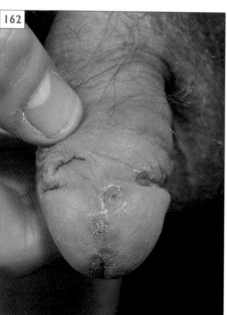

162 Primary syphilis (chancre). There is a painless, indurated nodule on the glans penis. This lesion had been ulcerated.

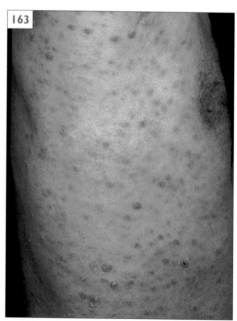

163 Secondary syphilis. An eruption of multiple red papules and plaques on the torso, some showing mild scaling.

known as 'snail-track' ulcers. Condylomata lata are flat, fleshy, papillomatous lesions of secondary syphilis occurring around the anus, scrotum, and vulva. Secondary syphilis is accompanied by constitutional symptoms (see below) which are worse at night.

DIFFERENTIAL DIAGNOSIS
Primary syphilis
Chancre:
- Herpes simplex virus infection (p. 142, grouped vesicles preceded by localized pain).
- Chancroid (tender, ulcerated papule caused by *Haemophilus ducreyi*).
- Granuloma inguinale (painless genital ulcer caused by *Calymmatobacterium granulomatis*).

Secondary syphilis
Maculo-papular syphilis:
- Pityriasis rosea (p. 38, eruption of oval, scaly patches following initial herald patch).
- Guttae psoriasis (p. 26, scaly plaques in symmetrical distribution, typical nail changes).
- Lichen planus (p. 36, violaceous papules and plaques, typical changes in mouth).
- Drug-induced exanthem (p. 220, widespread eruption of morbilliform erythema).
- Viral exanthem (p. 140, widespread eruption of morbilliform erythema).

Condylomata lata:
- Seborrhoeic keratosis (flat-topped keratotic plaque, often pigmented).
- Viral wart (skin-coloured papillomatous lesion).

164 Secondary syphilis. There are multiple red macules on the palms. Palmo-plantar skin is commonly involved in secondary syphilis.

165 Secondary syphilis. Close-up of palmar involvement showing discrete red macules with some scaling and desquamation.

COMPLICATIONS

Primary syphilis:

- Lymphadenopathy.

Secondary syphilis:

- Flu-like illness.
- Headache.
- Fever and weight loss.
- Lymphadenopathy.
- Hepatosplenomegaly.
- Bone pain (felt especially in the shins).

INVESTIGATIONS

- Blood count, basic chemistry, liver function tests (transaminases are often elevated in secondary syphilis).
- ESR, CRP (raised in secondary syphilis).
- Serum for nontreponemal tests: venereal disease reference laboratory test (VDRL), rapid plasma reagin test (RPR). VDRL and RPR are not positive until 1–4 weeks after the appearance of the chancre. Titres of VDRL and RPR are highest in secondary syphilis and can be used in assessing response to therapy. Nontreponemal tests may be negative in secondary syphilis with very high circulating antibodies (prozone effect). VDRL and RPR titres slowly decline and may become negative in late latent syphilis.
- Serum for treponemal antigen tests: *Treponema pallidum* haemagglutinin assay (TPHA), *Treponema pallidum* particle agglutination assay (TPPA). A positive VDRL or RPR should be confirmed with a TPHA test to differentiate a true-positive from a false-positive. Treponemal antigen tests remain positive for life.
- Dark-field examination of material from chancre or genital ulcer. Spirochaetes can be identified from chancres by dark-field microscopy confirming the diagnosis in primary syphilis before serological tests are positive.
- Skin biospy of secondary syphilis rash for histopathology (lymphoplasmacytic perivascular infiltrate).
- All patients with syphilis should be tested for HIV, gonorrhoea, and other sexually transmitted infections.

IMMEDIATE MANAGEMENT
Systemic therapy

- Primary and secondary syphilis should be treated with parenteral penicillin: **EITHER** IM procaine benzylpenicillin 600,000–900,000 U daily for 10 days **OR** IM benzathine penicillin 2.4 MU in a single dose.
- In penicillin-allergic patients give oral doxycycline 100 mg twice per day for 14 days.
- At-risk sexual contacts should be traced and offered relevant investigations and treatment.

LONG-TERM MANAGEMENT ISSUES

The cure rate for primary and secondary syphilis following correct antibiotic therapy is excellent. Following completion of treatment patients should receive clinical and serological follow-up at 3, 6, and 12 months. If untreated, secondary syphilis is followed by an asymptomatic stage with no clinical features but positive serology. This latent period may persist, be interrupted by a secondary stage relapse, or progress to the tertiary stage. Pregnant women who develop secondary syphilis and are untreated can infect their fetus resulting in congenital syphilis. Tertiary syphilis can present in the skin with granulomatous nodules, psoriasiform plaques, and gummas. Most morbidity from late syphilis results from cardiovascular and neurological problems.

Viral diseases

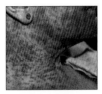 Viral
exanthem

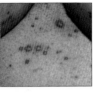 Chickenpox
(varicella)

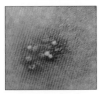 Herpes
simplex

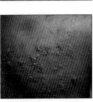 Herpes zoster
(shingles)

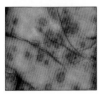 Erythema
multiforme

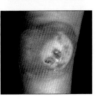 Orf

Viral exanthem

A systemic viral infection may be accompanied by a widespread eruption, termed an exanthem. Often the triggering virus remains unidentified but the combination of flu-like symptoms with a rash is suggestive of a viral aetiology.

CLINICAL FEATURES

Generally, an exanthem is distributed widely over the head, trunk, and limbs. Although the features can be nonspecific, certain infections produce a characteristic eruption:

- Infectious mononucleosis: there is fever, sore throat, and lymphadenopathy. Ten percent of patients will develop a morbilliform exanthem (**166**), however this increases to over 90% if ampicillin is taken during the illness.
- German measles (rubella): there is a 2 day prodrome of fever and coryza. The rash, which lasts for 2 days, is first noted on face and rapidly spreads to neck, arms, trunk, and legs. It consists of pink–red macules and papules which are discrete on the limbs but coalesce on the trunk.
- Measles (rubeola): there is a 3 day prodrome of fever, cough, coryza, and conjunctivitis. Koplik's spots are tiny white lesions which develop on the buccal mucosae 1–2 days before the exanthem. The rash starts behind the ears and on the forehead before spreading caudally over the entire body, reaching a peak at day 3 (**167**). It fades in a cephalocaudal manner over the next 2 days.
- Parvovirus B19: in children infection causes a 'slapped cheek' erythema. In adults, a proportion will develop a blotchy erythema on the extremities, termed 'papular, purpuric gloves-and-socks syndrome'.

Some viral exanthems have mucosal involvement (e.g. petechiae on the palate in EBV infection). Up to 75% of individuals with HIV seroconversion illness develop a maculopapular exanthem with predilection for the face, palms, and soles and accompanied, in some cases, by orogenital ulceration.

DIFFERENTIAL DIAGNOSIS

- Drug-induced exanthem (p. 220, a morbilliform eruption of pink macules on torso and limbs).
- Erythema multiforme (p. 144, urticated or blistered, target-like lesions especially on acral skin).
- Pityriasis rosea (p. 38, multiple oval lesions with a collarette of scale).
- Bacterial exanthem (*Streptococcus*-induced maculopapular exanthem).
- Acute graft-versus-host disease (p. 218, maculopapular exanthem with involvement of palms and soles).

COMPLICATIONS

Of all viral infections:
- Fever, malaise.
- Lymphadenopathy.
- Headache.
- Arthralgia and myalgia.

With infectious mononucleosis:
- Sore throat.
- Splenomegaly.
- Hepatitis.
- Meningoencephalilitis.
- Autoimmune haemolytic anaemia.

With measles:
- Pneumonitis.
- Hepatitis.
- Encephalitis.
- Thrombocytopenic purpura.

With German measles:
- Arthritis.
- Thrombocytopenic purpura.

With parvovirus B19:
- Transient aplastic crisis in patients with chronic haemolytic anaemia.

INVESTIGATIONS

- The diagnosis is usually made clinically.
- Blood count (atypical lymphocytosis in infectious mononucleosis).
- Basic chemistry, liver function tests (transient elevation of transaminases in infectious mononucleosis and measles).
- ESR, CRP (elevated CRP).

- Paul Bunnell test (positive in infectious mononucleosis).
- Serology for viral infections, including HIV, if suspected (a serum sample taken at the onset of the illness and then at recovery may show serological evidence of a specific viral infection).
- Skin biopsy for histopathology if diagnosis is in doubt (mild perivascular lymphocytic infiltrate).

IMMEDIATE MANAGEMENT
Topical therapy
- If mildly itchy, general emollient therapy.
- If very itchy, corticosteroid ointment, twice per day:
   face: mildly potent.
   trunk and limbs: moderately potent.

LONG-TERM MANAGEMENT ISSUES
Viral exanthems resolve spontaneously without long-term problems. Life-long immunity usually follows infection with viruses such as EBV, rubella, and measles. In many countries the MMR vaccination (mumps, measles, rubella) is given to infants at the age of 12–15 months and again at 4–6 years of age. A recent reduction in uptake of MMR has been accompanied by an increase in the number of adult cases of these infections. Following infectious mononucleosis some patients may develop a syndrome of prolonged fatigue.

166 Viral exanthem. There are numerous small, pink macules disseminated widely over the torso in this patient with infectious mononucleosis (EBV).

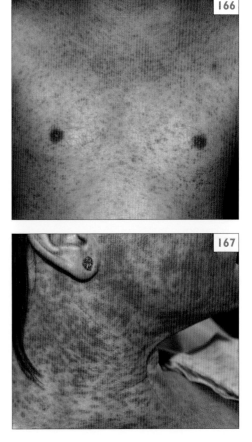

167 Viral exanthem. In this patient with measles there is a morbilliform exanthem of red macules which started on the face and neck.

Herpes simplex

Herpes simplex is a common viral infection affecting the skin and mucous membranes. Two sub-types are recognised: HSV1 is the main cause of oral and facial lesions, while HSV2 is responsible for the majority of genital infections. Both viruses persist in the sensory nerve ganglia after primary infection and can travel peripherally to the skin or mucous membranes to cause recurrent disease. HSV lesions are often painful and appear suddenly causing the patient to seek an urgent opinion.

CLINICAL FEATURES

Primary HSV1 infection usually occurs in childhood as stomatitis. Recurrent HSV1 infections occur most commonly on the face, particularly adjacent to the lips (herpes labialis), but can develop anywhere. Recurrent HSV infections are generally preceded by a short prodrome of burning or itching. The acute eruption consists of grouped vesicles on an inflamed base which become pustular and then crusted before healing within 7–10 days (**168, 169**). Recurrent HSV tends to recur in the same region but not always on the identical site. Primary HSV2 infection is generally encountered as a genital infection. It is characterized by painful vesicles and erosions on the penis or vulva which persist for 2–3 weeks before resolving. Episodes of recurrent genital herpes tend to be shorter in duration (**170**). Recurrent HSV2 infections may also manifest as clusters of vesicles on the buttocks. In the immunocompromised individual, HSV infection can become disseminated and cause a widespread eruption of vesicles, similar to chicken pox.

DIFFERENTIAL DIAGNOSIS
- Herpes zoster (p. 148, vesicles in a dermatomal distribution).
- Fixed drug eruption (p. 228, deep red circular patch, sometimes blisters, often on genital skin).
- Aphthous ulcers (common mouth ulcers which can be recurrent and multiple).

COMPLICATIONS
- Fever and malaise (especially with primary infections).
- Headache and myalgia (especially with primary infections).
- Regional painful lymphadenopathy (especially with primary infections).
- Erythema multiforme (occurs as a reaction to primary or recurrent infections).
- Bell's palsy.
- Encephalitis.

INVESTIGATIONS
- Swab of vesicle base for immuno-fluorescence and viral culture (for rapid confirmation of HSV infection immunofluorescence of vesicle scrapings can differentiate HSV1 and HSV2; culture of HSV from vesicle fluid takes 1–5 days; the most sensitive identification method is HSV detection and typing by PCR).
- Collection of vesicle fluid for electron microscopy (electron microscopy can rapidly identify viruses of the herpes family).
- Tzanck smear: scraping of the base of a vesicle on to a glass slide for cytology (demonstrates multinucleated giant cells and acidophilic intranuclear viral inclusion bodies in epithelial cells – a nonspecific test for cutaneous infection by a herpes virus).
- Skin swab for bacteriology if secondary infection suspected.

IMMEDIATE MANAGEMENT

Infection is usually self-limiting and often no treatment is necessary.

Topical therapy
- Topical aciclovir cream five times per day for 5 days may be effective if started early.

Systemic therapy
- If attacks are highly symptomatic: oral aciclovir can be given 200 mg five times per day for 5 days.

LONG-TERM MANAGEMENT ISSUES

Application of a sunblock to the lips can help reduce the frequency of UV-induced cold sores (herpes labialis) during the summer. Valaciclovir and famciclovir have better bioavailability and may be preferable to aciclovir if gastrointestinal absorption is a problem. Frequent, troublesome relapses can be halted with prophylactic treatment using aciclovir 400 mg twice per day or valaciclovir 500 mg once daily for 6 months. Condoms are effective in preventing HSV infection in genital herpes. Patients with persistent, relapsing HSV infections should be under the care of a dermatologist or genitourinary physician.

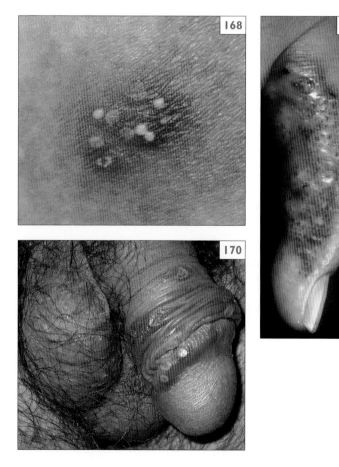

168 Herpes simplex. There is a cluster of tiny vesicles and vesico-pustules caused by reactivation of HSV1.

169 Herpetic whitlow. Numerous vesicles have coalesced along the side of the thumb producing a herpetic whitlow.

170 Genital herpes. There are several tiny ulcers with overlying slough on the glans, foreskin, and penile shaft. This was caused by reactivation of HSV2.

Erythema multiforme

Erythema multiforme (EM) is a distinctive eruption which occurs most commonly in response to an infection with HSV. EM is not a viral infection *per se*. Lesions of EM appear abruptly approximately 7 days after reactivation of either HSV1 or HSV2 infections. A proportion of cases occur in response to other infections (e.g. *Mycoplasma*, *Streptococcus*, orf) and to certain drugs (e.g. penicillin, sulphonamides, trimethoprim).

CLINICAL FEATURES
Some cases display purely cutaneous lesions, others exclusively mucosal involvement (especially if triggered by mycoplasma infections), however many patients have a mucocutaneous eruption involving acral and extensor surfaces of the limbs and the oral mucosae. Palms, soles, backs of hands, tops of feet, elbows, and knees are the commonest sites of EM. The constituent lesions take on a variety of forms (hence 'multiforme') but most are usually red circular macules or urticated papules. The most striking type of lesion is target-shaped and composed of concentric rings, the centre of which may become purpuric and blister (**171–173**). Oral lesions consist of blisters and ulcers (**174**). Skin involvement is usually asymptomatic but the mucosal lesions are often painful. Mucosal involvement of one site only is EM minor, whereas involvement of more than one site is termed EM major.

DIFFERENTIAL DIAGNOSIS
- Acute urticaria (p. 56, itchy weals, often displaying bizarre patterns).
- Urticarial vasculitis (p. 62, urticarial weals which are persistent).
- Chickenpox (p. 146, disseminated eruption of vesicles, each on a red macule).
- Stevens–Johnson syndrome (p. 230, mucocutaneous drug hypersensitivity syndrome with purpuric macules, target lesions, and blisters).
- Bullous pemphigoid (p. 66, itchy erythema with large tense blisters).

COMPLICATIONS
- Cervical lymphadenopathy (with oral lesions).

INVESTIGATIONS
- The diagnosis is usually made clinically.
- Swab of herpetic lesion for virology.
- Skin biopsy for histopathology (lymphocytic infiltrate at the dermoepidermal junction causing basal keratinocyte cell death with the presence of cytoid bodies; vesicular EM is characterized by a cleft at the dermoepidermal junction and extensive epidermal necrosis).

IMMEDIATE MANAGEMENT
Most cases are self-limiting, the lesions regressing within 2 weeks.

Topical therapy
- Corticosteroid ointment, twice per day: trunk and limbs: moderately potent or potent.
- Oral involvement may require anti-inflammatory and corticosteroid mouthwashes.
- Eye involvement needs scrupulous eye care, regular saline washes to remove crusts, and topical chloramphenicol.

Systemic therapy
- For severe oral ulceration or widespread skin involvement consider a short course of oral corticosteroids (e.g. prednisolone 0.5 mg/kg/day and reduce by 5 mg every 5th day).

LONG-TERM MANAGEMENT ISSUES
EM is often recurrent. Repeated episodes are usually associated with HSV reactivation. In these cases suppression of HSV reactivation with prophylactic antiherpetic therapy is usually indicated: aciclovir 400 mg twice per day or valaciclovir 500 mg once daily for 6 months. Patients with chronic, relapsing EM should be under the care of a dermatologist and may require second-line treatment with azathioprine.

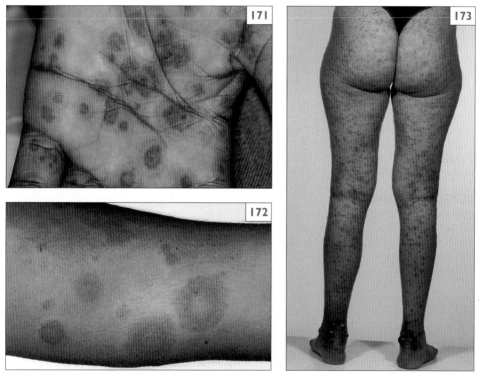

171 Erythema multiforme. The classical lesions of EM are target-like, comprising a series of alternating red and pale rings. The centre of each lesion is often dusky or blistered. In this patient the eruption was triggered by genital herpes.

172 Erythema multiforme. The concentric rings of erythema multiforme may be visible only on close examination. In this case the lesions appeared after an episode of genital herpes.

173 Erythema multiforme. This patient has extensive EM on the legs which appeared in association with a *Mycoplasma pneumoniae* chest infection. The lesions are blistering around the ankles.

174 Erythema multiforme. Involvement of the lower lip has produced an erosive cheilitis with haemorrhagic crusting.

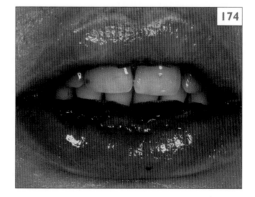

Chickenpox (varicella)

Chickenpox (varicella) is caused by primary infection with the varicella zoster virus. It is highly contagious and transmitted by droplet infection from the nasopharynx. Patients are infectious from 2 days before, to 5 days after the appearance of the rash. The incubation period is approximately 14 days. Less than 5% of all chickenpox cases occur in adults, however the disease tends to be more severe in this group and can result in life-threatening complications.

CLINICAL FEATURES

There is a short prodrome of fever, headache, myalgia, and malaise followed by the appearance of crops of red macules which rapidly develop into vesicles. The vesicles are surrounded by a zone of erythema (the areola) (**175**). With time the vesicles become pustular, crusted, and sometimes haemorrhagic (**176**). Typically lesions are seen at all stages of evolution. In adults, chickenpox lesions are often numerous and tend to involve the trunk, head, and proximal arms with relative sparing of the extremities (**177**). Vesicles are common in the mouth, especially on the palate. The eruption can be painful or itchy.

DIFFERENTIAL DIAGNOSIS

- Disseminated herpes simplex virus infection in the immunocompromised (p. 142, indistinguishable from chickenpox).
- Bullous impetigo (p. 118, areas of erythema with superficial blistering and honey-coloured crust).
- Erythema multiforme (p. 144, urticated or blistered target-like lesions especially on acral skin).

COMPLICATIONS

- Fever and malaise.
- Lymphadenopathy.
- Erysipelas, cellulitis.
- Pneumonitis (greatly increased in patients with chronic lung disease).
- Hepatitis.
- Myocarditis.
- Central nervous system involvement:
  - Encephalitis.
  - Polyradiculitis.
  - Myelitis.
- Fetal varicella syndrome.

INVESTIGATIONS

- The diagnosis is usually made clinically.
- Swab of vesicle base for immunofluorescence and viral culture (for rapid confirmation of VZV infection immunofluorescence of vesicle scrapings can differentiate VZV from HSV; culture of VZV from vesicle fluid takes 1–5 days; the most sensitive identification method is VZV detection by PCR).
- Collection of vesicle fluid for electron microscopy (electron microscopy can rapidly identify viruses of the herpes family).
- Tzanck smear: scraping of the base of a vesicle on to a glass slide for cytology (demonstrates multinucleated giant cells and acidophilic intranuclear viral inclusion bodies in epithelial cells – a nonspecific test for cutaneous infection by a herpes virus).
- Swab for bacterial culture (if secondary bacterial infection is suspected).
- Blood count, basic chemistry, liver function tests (if patient is systemically unwell).
- Chest radiography (if pneumonitis is suspected).

IMMEDIATE MANAGEMENT
Topical therapy
- Potassium permanganate soaks can be used for areas of vesiculation and crusting.

Systemic therapy
- The length of the illness can be reduced if oral medication is begun within the first 24 hr: aciclovir 800 mg 5 times per day or valaciclovir 1 g three times per day or famciclovir 500 mg three times per day, all for 7 days.
- Oral antibiotics for secondary bacterial infection.
- In immunocompromised patients, or for cases complicated by encephalitis or pneumonitis, give intravenous aciclovir 10 mg/kg three times per day for 7 days.

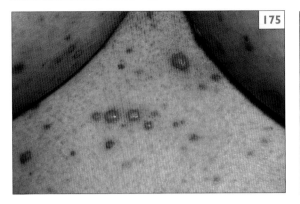

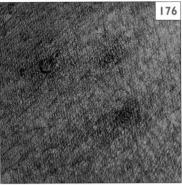

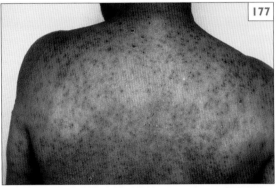

175 Chickenpox. Early chickenpox is characterized by discrete vesicles, each surrounded by a red flare.

176 Chickenpox. In later stages the vesicles burst to leave small erosions with an overlying haemorrhagic crust.

177 Chickenpox. In adults chickenpox is often extensive. Typically there are lesions in all stages of evolution.

Supportive therapy

- If the patient is systemically ill or deteriorates, admit to hospital for monitoring of vital signs, administration of intravenous therapy, and management of complications.

LONG-TERM MANAGEMENT ISSUES

Most individuals develop immunity after a single episode of chickenpox. Recurrences are rare, but can occasionally occur. In the first 28 weeks of pregnancy, primary maternal infection with VZV can result in the fetal varicella syndrome causing a wide range of congenital abnormalities (cicatricial skin lesions, limb hypoplasia, central nervous system and eye abnormalities). Nonimmune pregnant women who have contact with a case of chicken pox or shingles should receive specific varicella zoster immunoglobulin (VZIG). VZIG can also be given to any immunocompromised patient after contact with infective varicella. A varicella zoster vaccine is available.

Herpes zoster (shingles)

Herpes zoster, or shingles, is a localized, dermatomal eruption caused by reactivation of latent varicella zoster virus within the peripheral sensory nerves. The elderly and immunocompromised are particularly susceptible. In the immunocompromised herpes zoster is a significant disease and may be associated with severe side-effects including life-threatening visceral dissemination.

CLINICAL FEATURES

There is a prodrome of regional pain which precedes the appearance of herpes zoster by 1–3 days. The eruption is characterized by a one or more groups of red papules which evolve into vesicles. Groups of vesicles are located within one dermatome (**178**). With time the vesicles become confluent and form a distinctive unilateral, linear dermatosis which is confined by the dermatome and stops at the midline (**179**). The most common sites of

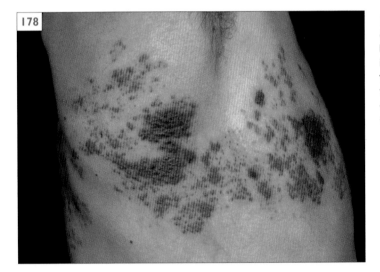

178 Herpes zoster (shingles). There is a broad band of inflamed vesicles which extends around the right side of the chest involving the T3 dermatome.

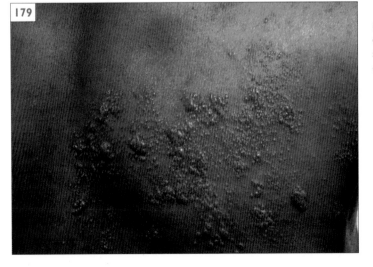

179 Herpes zoster (shingles). This picture of thoracic shingles shows the sharp cut-off at the midline.

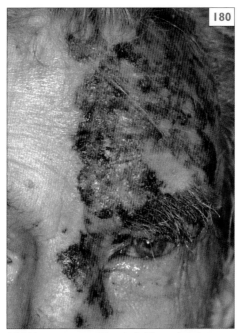

180 Herpes zoster (shingles). The ophthalmic branch of the left trigeminal nerve is involved (ophthalmic zoster). The eruption was associated with severe pain (herpetic neuralgia) which persisted for several months.

involvement are facial (ophthalmic branch of trigeminal nerve) (**180**) and mid-thoracic to upper lumbar dermatomes (T3–L2). Rupture of the vesicles will result in eroded areas. Very active infection may produce large blisters which can be haemorrhagic. Secondary bacterial infection is common, the vesicles becoming pustular and then crusted. Although one dermatome is usually affected, areas of secondary spread occur with vesicles found beyond the affected dermatome. Disseminated herpes zoster may develop in the immuno-compromised and is defined as more than 20 vesicles outside the primary and adjacent dermatomes. Following cutaneous dissemination systemic involvement (liver, lungs, brain) occurs in up to 10% of these at-risk patients.

DIFFERENTIAL DIAGNOSIS
- Herpes simplex (p. 142, a cluster of vesicles on a red base).
- Bullous impetigo (p. 118, areas of erythema with superficial blistering and honey-coloured crust).
- Erythema multiforme (p. 144, urticated or blistered target-like lesions especially on acral skin).
- Allergic contact dermatitis (p. 18, eczema in a localized area or unusual distribution).

COMPLICATIONS

- Fever, headache, and malaise.
- Lymphadenopathy.
- Post-herpetic neuralgia.
- Ocular complications (with ophthalmic zoster):
  - Eyelid scarring.
  - Keratitis.
  - Scleritis.
  - Uveitis.
  - Panophthalmitis.
- Ramsey-Hunt syndrome (facial palsy with ipsilateral lesions on external ear, tympanic membrane or anterior two-thirds of tongue).
- Systemic VZV infection (pneumonitis, encephalitis, hepatitis, myocarditis).

INVESTIGATIONS

- The diagnosis is usually made clinically.
- Swab of vesicle base for immunofluorescence and viral culture (for rapid confirmation of VZV infection immunofluorescence of vesicle scrapings can differentiate VZV from HSV; culture of VZV from vesicle fluid takes 1–5 days; the most sensitive identification method is VZV detection by PCR).
- Collection of vesicle fluid for electron microscopy (electron microscopy can rapidly identify viruses of the herpes family).
- Tzanck smear: scraping of the base of a vesicle on to a glass slide for cytology (demonstrates multinucleated giant cells and acidophilic intranuclear viral inclusion bodies in epithelial cells – a nonspecific test for cutaneous infection by a herpes virus).
- Swab for bacterial culture (if secondary bacterial infection is suspected).
- Blood count, basic chemistry, liver function tests (if patient is systemically unwell).
- Investigations for immunosuppression (if considered): immunoglobulins and electrophoresis, T cell subsets, HIV test.
- Chest radiograph (with disseminated shingles).

IMMEDIATE MANAGEMENT
Topical therapy

- Potassium permanganate soaks to areas of vesiculation or crusting.

Systemic therapy

- The severity of post-herpetic neuralgia may be reduced if active therapy is instituted early (within 72 hr of first vesicle): aciclovir 800 mg 5 times per day or valaciclovir 1 g three times per day or famciclovir 500 mg three times per day, all for 7 days.
- Patients will require adequate analgesia.
- Oral antibiotics for secondary bacterial infection.
- In immunocompromised patients, or for cases complicated by encephalitis or pneumonitis, give intravenous aciclovir 10 mg/kg three times per day for 7 days.

Supportive therapy

- If the patient is systemically ill or deteriorates admit to hospital for monitoring of vital signs, administration of intravenous therapy, and management of complications.

LONG-TERM MANAGEMENT ISSUES

Post-herpetic neuralgia (PHN) affects 50% of patients who are older than 60 years. There is a particularly high rate of PHN following ophthalmic zoster. Usually PHN settles within 6 months, however patients may require pain relief with drugs such as amitriptyline or gabapentin. Topical capsaicin cream can also be helpful. Extensive herpes zoster, especially in the immunocompromised, may be complicated by cutaneous necrosis with delayed healing and scarring. A patient with ophthalmic zoster should be under the care of an ophthalmologist to monitor potential ocular complications such as impaired corneal sensation, secondary bacterial infection, and scarring.

Orf

Orf is caused by a parapox virus which infects young sheep and goats. In humans orf occurs mainly as an occupational disease in individuals who handle these animals (e.g. farmers and butchers). Direct inoculation from an infected source into the skin usually produces the inflammatory lesion, however orf can also be transmitted via fomites.

CLINICAL FEATURES

The initial lesion is a small, firm, red or violaceous papule which gradually enlarges (**181**). In established orf a target appearance may occur with a central area of erythema surrounded by concentric white and red rings. Haemorrhagic, pustular, or bullous lesions may also occur. With time, the typical nodule becomes necrotic and develops a crusted, umbilicated centre, growing to 1–3 cm before gradually regressing. The lesions are often painful and may also be itchy.

DIFFERENTIAL DIAGNOSIS

- Furunculosis (p. 120, an abscess arising from an infected hair follicle).
- Pyogenic granuloma (p. 191, a rapidly-growing vascular nodule which bleeds easily).
- Giant molluscum contagiosum (skin-coloured umbilicated nodule).
- Keratoacanthoma (p. 188, dome-shaped nodule with central keratin plug).

COMPLICATIONS

- Regional lymphadenopathy.
- Lymphangitis.
- Fever.
- Erythema multiforme.

INVESTIGATIONS

- The diagnosis is usually made clinically.
- Skin biopsy for histopathology (oedema of the epidermis with vacuolization and balloon degeneration, cytoplasmic inclusion bodies are seen; a prominent inflammatory infiltrate in the dermis).

IMMEDIATE MANAGEMENT

Treatment is often not necessary: orf will clear spontaneously within 6 weeks.

Systemic therapy

- Oral antibiotics if there is secondary bacterial infection.
- Adequate analgesia.

LONG-TERM MANAGEMENT ISSUES

There is little long-term morbidity.

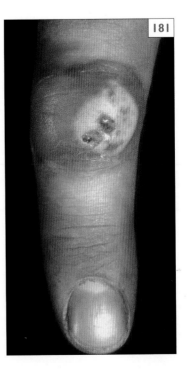

181 Orf. There is a large inflamed nodule on the dorsal aspect of the forefinger, a typical site. The white central zone indicates a site of previous blistering.

Fungal diseases

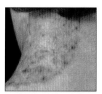

Tinea (dermatophyte infections)

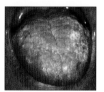

Candidiasis

Tinea (dermatophyte infections)

Dermatophytes are fungi capable of causing skin infections of the type known as tinea or ringworm. The clinical features result from a combination of keratin destruction and an inflammatory host response. The lesions of tinea tend to develop slowly but the associated itch is often intense and provokes the patient to seek an urgent opinion.

CLINICAL FEATURES

A common clinical characteristic of dermatophyte infections is the presence of an itchy red patch with an expanding margin.

- Tinea corporis (body): disc-like or annular lesion(s) with a scaly raised edge (**182, 183**). Often seen on the torso or arms, occasionally the face (tinea facei). If untreated the patch may grow to be many centimetres in diameter.
- Tinea cruris (groins and other flexures): a red patch with an active, advancing margin extending from the groin to the inner thigh, natal cleft or perineum (**184**).
- Tinea pedis (foot): usually characterized by peeling and maceration of the lateral toe clefts, sometimes extending on to the soles (**185**). Occasionally there is blistering (usually with infection by *Trichophyton interdigitale*). 'Mocassin'-type tinea pedis can involve the whole of the plantar surface, with white scaling on a pink background, seen most usually with *T. rubrum* infection.
- Tinea capitis (scalp): this is rare in adults. There are patches of hair loss with oedema, scaling, and sometimes pustules (**186**). There is associated itching and sometimes cervical lymphadenopathy.

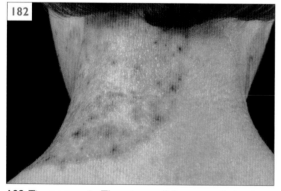

182 Tinea corporis. There is a well demarcated, circular, red patch with mild scaling.

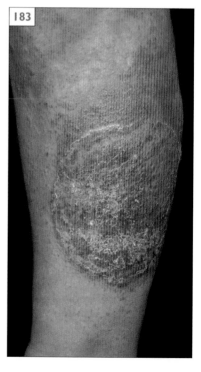

183 Tinea corporis. In this case the red, circular patch of tinea is surrounded by a zone of acute inflammation.

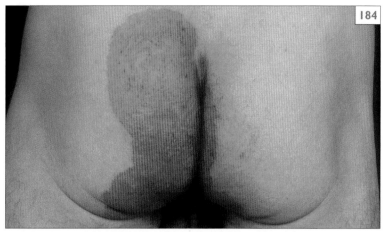

184 Tinea cruris. A well demarcated, red patch is extending from the natal cleft. Tinea cruris also involves the groins.

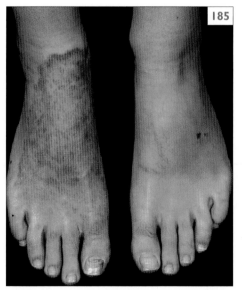

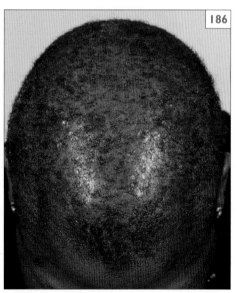

185 Tinea pedis. Confluent involvement over the dorsum of the right foot with an active, scaly margin. There is also onychomycosis of the great toenail.

186 Tinea capitis. Erythema of the scalp with patchy alopecia.

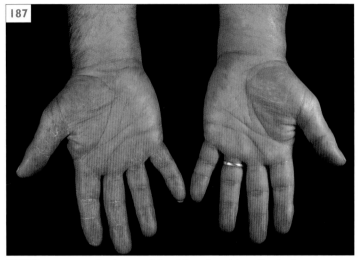

187 Tinea manum. Erythema of the right palm with scaling in the creases.

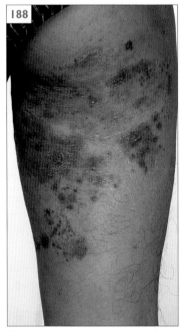

188 Tinea incognito. A poorly defined zone of erythema on the posterior thigh containing papules and pustules.

- Tinea manum (hand): diffuse fine scaling of the palmar skin with accentuation of the creases. Usually only one palm is involved (**187**).
- Tinea incognito: this results from the inappropriate application of potent topical steroid to a dermatophyte infection which alters the physical signs. Pustules and papules are present but there is loss of the usual scaling and annular rim (**188**).
- Tinea unguum (or onychomycosis): this is a chronic dermatophyte nail infection causing a dystrophic, thickened nail plate with white, yellow or dark discolouration and subungual hyperkeratosis (**185**).

DIFFERENTIAL DIAGNOSIS
Tinea corporis
- Psoriasis (p. 28, scaly plaques in a symmetrical distribution, typical nail changes).
- Pityriasis rosea (p. 38, an eruption of slightly scaly patches following an initial 'herald' lesion).
- Mycosis fungoides (p. 194, pink–red patches with superficial atrophy, distributed asymmetrically).

Tinea cruris
- Flexural psoriasis (p. 28, symmetrical, red, patches in flexures with well demarcated margins).
- Candidiasis (p. 158, shiny red patches in flexures with tiny superficial pustules and satellite lesions).
- Erythrasma (corynebacterial infection causing red–brown patches in flexures).

Tinea pedis/manum
- Palmo-plantar psoriasis (p. 30, scaling and well demarcated erythema).
- Pompholyx eczema (p. 12, vesicles with dryness, scaling, and redness).

Tinea capitis
- Psoriasis (p. 28, well demarcated scaly plaques, involvement of the hairline).
- Seborrheoic dermatitis (p. 20, diffuse scalp redness and dandruff).

Tinea incognito
- Bacterial folliculitis (p. 120, follicular pustules and papules).
- Discoid eczema (p. 14, well circumscribed patch of dermatitis).

COMPLICATIONS
Tinea pedis can act as a portal of entry for bacterial infection leading to cellulitis.

INVESTIGATIONS
- Mycology samples (microscopy and culture):
- Tinea corporis/cruris/pedis/manum: skin scrapings.
- Tinea capitis: plucked hairs, scrapings, and brushings.
- Onychomycosis: nail clippings.
- Microscopy of a potassium hydroxide preparation will reveal fungal hyphae. Appropriate culture will confirm the presence of pathogenic fungi and identify the species of dermatophyte.

IMMEDIATE MANAGEMENT
Topical therapy
For limited tinea corporis, tinea cruris, tinea pedis, and tinea manum treat topically:
- EITHER an allylamine-derivative cream twice per day for 2–3 weeks (e.g. terbinafine).
- OR an azole cream twice per day for 2–3 weeks (e.g. clotrimazole).

Systemic therapy
Oral therapy is needed in tinea corporis with multiple sites of involvement, extensive tinea cruris, 'moccasin'-type tinea pedis and tinea capitis:
- Terbinafine 250 mg once daily for 4 weeks.

If oral terbinafine is contraindicated, use oral itraconazole:
- For tinea corporis and tinea cruris, itraconazole 100 mg once daily for 15 days.
- For tinea pedis and tinea manum, itraconazole 100 mg once daily for 30 days or 200 mg twice daily for 7 days.

For onychomycosis oral therapy is usually necessary:
Fingernails:
- Terbinafine 250 mg once daily for 6 weeks.
- OR itraconazole 200 mg once daily for 3 months.
- OR itraconazole 400 mg once daily for 1 week, and thereafter given for 1 week each month for 2–3 months.

Toenails:
- Terbinafine 250 mg once daily for 3 months.
- OR itraconazole 400 mg once daily for 1 week, and thereafter given for 1 week each month for 3–4 months.

LONG-TERM MANAGEMENT ISSUES
Dermatophyte infections are contagious through direct physical contact. Other family members should be examined. In a patient with a dermatophyte infection on the skin look for fingernail or toenail involvement and treat as above.

Candidiasis

The cutaneous and mucosal manifestations of candidiasis can be separated into a number of clinical disorders each characterized by the site of involvement. Oral candidiasis occurs in the immunosuppressed, the elderly (especially those wearing dentures), and in patients taking inhaled or systemic corticosteroids. Vulvo-vaginal candidiasis is extemely common in normal adult women. Cutaneous infection most commonly causes an intertrigo (inflam-mation affecting the skin folds) but may also be implicated in balanitis, folliculitis, paronychia, and in an occlusion dermatosis on the backs of bed-ridden patients. Generally, invasion by *Candida* relies on an underlying host impair-ment which may be a local epithelial problem or due to reduced immunity, such as that asso-ciated with immunosuppressive drugs, HIV infection or diabetes mellitus.

CLINICAL FEATURES

- Oral candidiasis: there are white plaques on inflamed oral mucosae (**189**) which may appear red and glazed (acute erythematous candidiasis). The mouth may be sore.
- Vulvovaginal candidiasis: there is vulval redness, oedema, white plaques, and a watery or 'cottage cheese' discharge. Itching is usual. Vaginal pain and dyspareunia may also occur.
- Candida intertrigo: this tends to occur in macerated skin of the groins, axillae, submammary folds, and the natal cleft. The eruption is itchy and sore and starts as a moist erythema deep in the fold. Subsequently candida intertrigo spreads beyond the area of contact, the edge being irregular and surmounted by superficial pustules. Beyond the margin, satellite red papules or pustules may be seen (**190**). The pustules in candidiasis tend to rupture giving rise to erosions and a collarette of scale.
- Cutaneous candidiasis: in areas of occlusion, such as the skin of the back or under dressings, *Candida* colonization can cause a vesicopustular reaction or folliculitis.

- Candidal paronychia: this occurs in individuals who are perpetually involved in wet work (e.g. bartenders, hairdressers). Typically there is redness, swelling, and tenderness of the nail fold with retraction of the cuticle. Occasionally pus can be expressed.

DIFFERENTIAL DIAGNOSIS
Oral candidiasis
- Lichen planus (p. 36, network of white lines on buccal mucosae).

Vulvovaginal candidiasis
- Contact dermatitis (p. 18, itchy erythema with lichenification).

Candida intertrigo
- Tinea cruris (p. 154, a unilateral itchy, red patch with an advancing margin).
- Seborrhoeic dermatitis (p. 20, itchy erythema in flexures).
- Flexural psoriasis (symmetrical, red, patches in flexures with well demarcated margins).

Cutaneous candidiasis
- Cutaneous aspergillosis (pustules and erythema, usually in the immunocompromised).
- Generalized pustular psoriasis (p. 32, widespread erythema with waves of superficial pustules).
- Acute generalized exanthematous pustulosis (p. 226, widespread pustular drug eruption).

Candidal paronychia
- Bacterial paronychia (painful erythema and collection of pus at nail fold).
- Herpetic whitlow (p. 142, painful cluster of vesicles along finger margin).

COMPLICATIONS
- Systemic candidiasis.

INVESTIGATIONS
- Scraping or swab for microbiology.
- Serum glucose (to exclude diabetes).
- Blood count (to exclude leucopenia).

IMMEDIATE MANAGEMENT

- Oral candidiasis: nystatin lozenges or suspension twice per day for 1–2 weeks. Dentures should be removed overnight and cleaned with saline before they are replaced. In immunocompromised patients use oral fluconazole 50 mg once daily for 7–14 days or itraconazole 100 mg once daily for 15 days.
- Vulvovaginal candidiasis: EITHER clotrimazole pessaries 200 mg once daily for 3 nights, OR oral therapy with fluconazole 150 mg as a single dose or itraconazole 400 mg as a single dose.
- Candida intertrigo: clotrimazole cream 1% twice daily for 1–2 weeks. If extensive, fluconazole 150 mg as a single dose. Keep macerated skin folds clean and dry.
- Cutaneous candidiasis: clotrimazole cream 1% twice daily for 1–2 weeks. If extensive, fluconazole 150 mg as a single dose. Keep affected skin clean and dry.
- Candida paronychia: clotrimazole solution 1% to the affected nail fold(s) twice per day for 3 months.

LONG-TERM MANAGEMENT ISSUES

In relapsing vaginal candidiasis confirm that recurring symptoms are accompanied by *Candida* infection by repeating swabs. Longer-term therapy with a course of oral fluconazole or itraconazole over 2–3 weeks followed by topical therapy with clotrimazole may be helpful. Chronic mucocutaneous candidiasis is usually seen in children but can occur with an adult onset. It tends to occur in association with either thymoma or SLE.

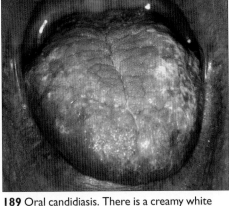

189 Oral candidiasis. There is a creamy white coating on the tongue. This patient was receiving oral corticosteroids.

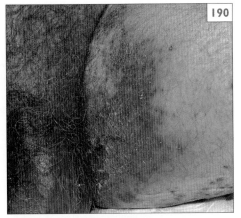

190 Flexural candidiasis. There is erythema in the fold of the groin with pustules at the margin and satellite pustules beyond the margin.

Dermatoses caused by arthropods

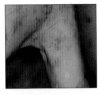

Scabies

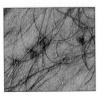

Insect bites

Pediculosis (lice)

Scabies

Infestation by the *Sarcoptes scabiei* mite causes scabies which is characterized, in most cases, by an intense and distressing itch. The mite is transmitted by direct physical contact from an infested individual. Thereafter the female burrows into the skin and lays her eggs in the stratum corneum of the epidermis. Scabies results from sensitization to the mites and their faeces. The diagnosis should be considered in an individual developing severe, widespread itching, particularly if there are family members or close contacts who are also itchy.

CLINICAL FEATURES

There is severe and generalized pruritus, particularly bad at night, and an eruption of patchy erythema, papules, and excoriations (**191**). Burrows are pathognomic and appear as small, scaly, linear lesions found at the wrists, sides of fingers, finger web spaces (**192**), and the insteps of the feet. A burrow is the width of a human hair, 2–10 mm long and the female mite may be seen as a tiny black dot at the distal end of it. The mite can be visualized better using a dermatoscope. Excoriated papules are often grouped around the axillae, periumbilical region, buttocks, and thighs. Larger, inflammatory nodules are found on the male genitalia (**193**), at the waist, and on the buttocks. In crusted (Norwegian) scabies the patient, who is usually elderly or immunosuppressed, is infested by vast numbers of mites and has a widespread, scaly dermatosis, which is often asymptomatic (**194, 195**).

DIFFERENTIAL DIAGNOSIS

- Atopic dermatitis (p. 8, flexural eczema as part of the atopic diathesis).
- Pompholyx eczema (p. 12, vesicular eczema on palmo-plantar skin).
- Dermatitis herpetiformis (p. 72, itchy vesicles on buttocks and elbows).
- Pediculosis corporis (p. 166, body lice causing bites and excoriations at sites of clothing seams).

COMPLICATIONS

- Secondary bacterial infection (rarely glomerulonephritis can complicate secondary streptococcal infection of scabies).

INVESTIGATIONS

- The diagnosis is usually made clinically.
- The mite can be extracted from a burrow on the tip of a blunt needle and visualized microscopically.
- Scrapings from burrows, subsequently exposed to 10% potassium hydroxide (KOH) solution and viewed microscopically, may reveal mites or eggs.

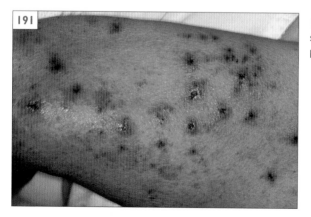

191 Scabies. The scratching of scabetic itch can produce prurigo papules and nodules.

192 Scabies. A number of tiny, linear, scaly lesions (burrows) are seen in this finger web.

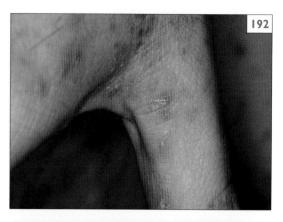

193 Scabies. Inflamed nodules on the shaft of the penis and scrotum are characteristic of scabies.

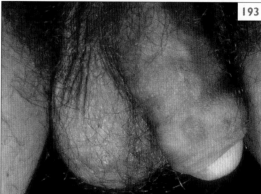

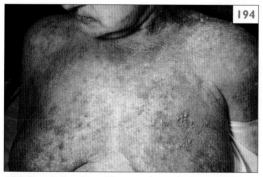

194 Crusted scabies. This patient with dementia had a widespread scaly dermatosis. A sample of the scale was teeming with scabetic mites.

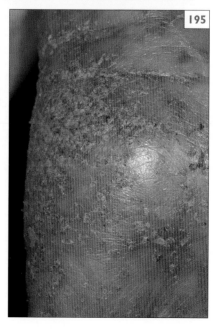

195 Crusted scabies. In crusted scabies there is adherent scale and background erythema.

IMMEDIATE MANAGEMENT
Topical therapy
- 5% permethrin cream or 0.5% malathion lotion is applied to all skin below the neck. This should include the genitals, soles of feet, between the digits, and under the nails. It must be left on for at least 12 hours before being washed off. The treatment should be repeated 1 week later.
- Close personal and household contacts should also be treated, regardless of symptoms.
- General emollient therapy; aqueous cream containing 1% menthol can be soothing.
- Corticosteroid ointment, twice per day (can help the itch once antiscabetic treatment has been administered):
     trunk and limbs: moderately potent.
- Crotamiton cream is a useful antipruritic agent.

Systemic therapy
- A sedating antihistamine taken at night will help the itch (e.g. hydroxyzine 25–50 mg).
- In crusted (Norwegian) scabies, or nonresponding scabies, two doses of oral ivermectin 200 μg/kg 7 days apart will eradicate the infestation. Avoid ivermectin in pregnant women and infants.

LONG-TERM MANAGEMENT ISSUES
Despite effective mite eradication residual itching commonly persists for a few weeks. Reassure the patient that it will resolve. If, however, the patient continues to develop new burrows it is important to repeat antiscabetic therapy and to trace and treat any close contacts. Symptomatic scabetic nodules can persist for a number of months after the infestation has been eradicated. Intralesional steroid and cryotherapy can be used to treat these lesions.

Insect bites

Insect bites are extremely common during the summer months and are usually acquired from flying arthropods found in gardens or in the countryside. Midges and mosquitoes are commonly encountered biting (blood-sucking) insects; mosquitoes are found near water, including ponds and ditches, and feed between dusk and dawn. Sometimes the source of an insect bite can be difficult to trace. In these patients it is important to consider other aspects in the history which may point to insect exposure: for example, contact with a pet infested by an arthropod (such as *Cheyletiella*), a move to a new home with infested soft furnishings, or sleeping in a bed infested by bed bugs. Bite reactions cause significant symptoms if the patient's immunological response is excessive or if there are numerous lesions. Patients with an underlying lymphoproliferative disorder (e.g. chronic lymphocytic leukaemia) may develop florid insect bite reactions.

CLINICAL FEATURES
An itchy, urticated papule develops initially at the site of the bite which subsequently evolves into a firm nodule often surmounted by a central vesicle or haemorrhagic punctum (**196**). Lesions tend to be in clusters of three or four, appearing in lines or groups. The bite reaction usually persists for several days before resolving without scarring. Lichenification and secondary eczema may alter the clinical picture. In a severe insect bite reaction large blisters may develop (**197**). Bed bugs can produce florid reactions; purpuric macules occur in the nonsensitized individual, large itchy weals with haemorrhagic puncta in sensitized subjects.

DIFFERENTIAL DIAGNOSIS
- Atopic prurigo (itchy papules and flexural eczema as part of the atopic diathesis).
- Scabies (p. 162, generalized itching with burrows in the finger webs and at the wrists).
- Dermatitis herpetiformis (p. 72, itchy vesicles on buttocks and elbows).
- Bullous pemphigoid (p. 66, itchy erythema with large, tense blisters).
- Urticarial vasculitis (p. 62, itchy or burning weals which are persistent).

COMPLICATIONS
- Secondary bacterial infection.
- Fever and malaise (if the bites are numerous).

INVESTIGATIONS
- The diagnosis is usually made clinically.
- Skin biopsy for histopathology if diagnosis is in doubt (oedema in the papillary dermis and a perivascular inflammatory infiltrate with eosinophils).

IMMEDIATE MANAGEMENT
Topical therapy
- Corticosteroid ointment, twice per day:
  - face: mildly potent.
  - trunk and limbs: potent.

Systemic therapy
- An oral antihistamine will ease the itch.
- Secondary bacterial infection may require oral antibiotics.

LONG-TERM MANAGEMENT ISSUES
The use of an insect repellent (50% N, N-diethyl-meta-toluamide (DEET)) may be helpful. If possible, the source of the bites must be traced and eradicated. Infested domestic pets should be treated by a vet. An infested home may require insecticidal treatment from an appropriate environmental pest control agency.

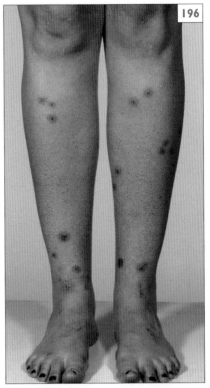

196 Insect bites. Numerous grouped nodules each with a central, haemorrhagic punctum.

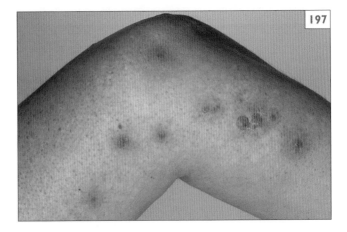

197 Insect bites. A line of bullous insect bites on a leg.

Pediculosis (lice)

Lice are wingless insects which are obligate human parasites: *Pediculosis humanus capitis* is the head louse, *P. humanus humanus* is the body louse, and *Phthirus pubis* is the pubic louse. All have claws adapted to clinging to hair and are able to cement their eggs to hair shafts or clothing. Head lice are spread by head-to-head contact, body lice are transmitted via infested bedding or clothing, and pubic lice are spread by sexual contact.

CLINICAL FEATURES

In head lice (pediculosis capitis) there is initial itching of the sides and back of the scalp and then generalized scalp pruritus. Examination reveals multiple white 'nits' (egg cases) stuck on the hair shafts (**198**). The head louse, which is usually hard to find, measures approximately 3 mm in length. Persistent scratching may result in secondary infection of the scalp and cervical lymphadenopathy. There are often pruritic papules on the back of the neck and shoulders (**199**). Sometimes a widespread hypersensitivity rash, or pediculid, develops on the torso and limbs.

In body lice (pediculosis corporis) the patient complains of generalized pruritus, especially severe on the trunk. The patient is usually unkempt and shows signs of self-neglect. Examination reveals bites and excoriations usually most marked at the sites of clothing seams (**200**). If it is allowed to persist the eruption resembles chronic eczema. Inspection of the clothing will reveal eggs in the seams.

In pubic lice (pediculosis pubis) there is severe itching in the pubic area, nits will be visible on the pubic hair, and bites may be seen on the pubic skin (**201**). Blue–grey macules on the lower abdomen and thighs are also secondary to bites. Eczematization and secondary infection of the pubic skin may follow. Pubic lice can also be found on facial hair, including eyelashes (**202**).

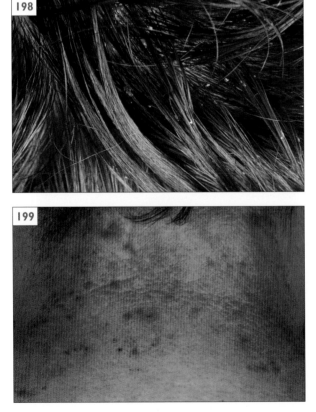

198 Head lice (pediculosis capitis). Several white 'nits' (egg cases) are adherent to the hair shafts. A louse is also visible.

199 Head lice (pediculosis capitis). Pruritic papules with erythema on the posterior neck are typical in head lice.

200 Body lice (pediculosis corporis). Excoriations and lichenification occur at the site of contact between the seams of infested clothing and the skin.

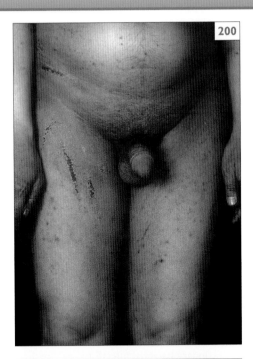

201 Pubic lice (pediculosis pubis). A number of lice can be seen adhering to the pubic hair.

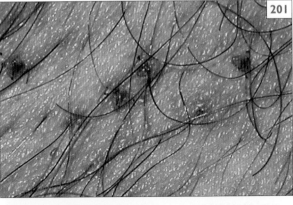

202 Pubic lice (pediculosis pubis). Pubic lice can also be found on the eyelashes.

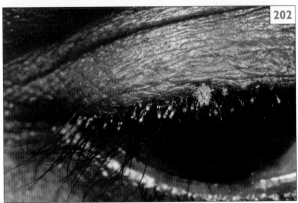

DIFFERENTIAL DIAGNOSIS
Head lice
- Seborrhoeic dermatitis (p. 20, erythema and scaling of the scalp, face, and chest).
- Tinea capitis (p. 154, well circumscribed area of erythema and scaling on the scalp).

Body lice
- Scabies (p. 162, generalized itching with burrows, usually in finger webs and at wrists).
- Atopic dermatitis (p. 8, flexural eczema as part of the atopic diathesis).

Pubic lice
- Scabies (p. 162, generalized itching with burrows in finger webs and wrists, nodules on genital skin).
- Contact dermatitis (p. 18, eczema in a localized area or unusual distribution).

COMPLICATIONS
- Lymphadenopathy.
- Secondary bacterial infection.
- *Bartonella* infections (body lice are vectors for relapsing fever, urban trench fever caused by *B. quintana*, and epidemic typhus: these rare diseases may be seen in refugees from natural disasters or war).

INVESTIGATIONS
- The diagnosis is usually made clinically.
- In the case of pediculosis pubis screen for other sexually transmitted diseases (herpes, warts, syphilis, gonorrhoea, *Chlamydia*, trichomoniasis, and HIV).

IMMEDIATE MANAGEMENT
Topical therapy
Head lice:
- 5% permethrin cream or cream rinse should be applied to the hair and left on for 12 hr. The treatment should be repeated 1 week later. 0.5% malathion lotion (aqueous basis) can be used as a second-line agent.
- Wet combing of the hair with a fine-toothed comb will mechanically remove lice and nits. Wet combing needs to be repeated every 3 days for 2 weeks.

Body lice:
- Infested clothing and bedding must be washed at high temperature to kill the lice.
- General emollient therapy; aqueous cream containing 1% menthol can be soothing.
- Corticosteroid ointment, twice per day: trunk and limbs: moderately potent.
- Crotamiton cream is a useful antipruritic agent.

Pubic lice:
- Apply 5% permethrin cream or 0.5% malathion lotion (aqueous basis) to all skin surfaces, including scalp and face, with attention to beard and eyebrows. Wash off after 12 hr. Repeat after 7 days. For infested eyelashes, use white soft paraffin ointment.
- The patient should launder clothing and bedding and avoid sexual contact until the infestation is eradicated.

LONG-TERM MANAGEMENT ISSUES
Therapeutic failure may result from continued contact with an infested individual or the presence of drug resistance. The continued use of pediculicides can cause resistance and therefore temporary withdrawal of certain agents may be deemed necessary.

Travellers' and tropical dermatoses

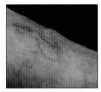 Cutaneous larva migrans

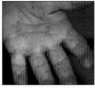 Rickettsial spotted fevers

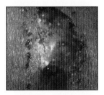 Furuncular myiasis

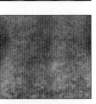 Dengue

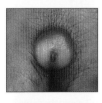 Tungiasis

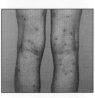 Swimmer's itch

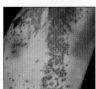 Leishmaniasis

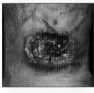 Sea-bathers' eruption

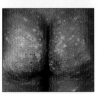 Onchocerciasis

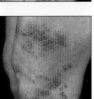 Jellyfish stings

Sporotrichosis

Cutaneous larva migrans

Cutaneous larva migrans results from invasion of the skin with the larvae of animal hookworms. The most frequent causative organism is the larva of the dog hookworm, *Ancylostoma braz14iliensis*, which is deposited on the ground from faeces of infected dogs and cats. Human infection is usually acquired from walking, sitting, or lying on contaminated beaches in the Caribbean, Central and South America, Africa, Southeast Asia, and southeastern USA.

CLINICAL FEATURES

Cutaneous larva migrans is found at sites of larva penetration, often the sole of the foot or on the buttocks. The typical lesion is a solitary, red, serpiginous track, which is very itchy (**203**). Vesicular areas may occur. The track extends gradually, progressing at a rate of a few millimetres per day. If large numbers of larvae are involved several tracks may be visible (**204**) or if scratching has been intense the characteristic signs may be obscured.

DIFFERENTIAL DIAGNOSIS

- Tinea incognito (p. 154, localized erythema, papules, and pustules).
- Contact dermatitis (p. 18, eczema in a localized area or unusual distribution).

COMPLICATIONS

- Regional lymphadenopathy (with secondary bacterial infection).
- Lymphangitis (with secondary bacterial infection).
- Erysipelas/cellulitis (with secondary bacterial infection).
- Pulmonary eosinophilia of Loeffler's syndrome (associated with severe infestations).

INVESTIGATIONS

- The diagnosis is usually made clinically.
- Swab for bacteriology (if secondary infection is suspected).

IMMEDIATE MANAGEMENT
Topical therapy

- Cryotherapy to the larva (situated in front of the leading end of the track).
- Topical 10% thiobendazole

Systemic therapy

Use systemic therapy if cryotherapy is ineffective or topical thiobendazole is unobtainable:

- Oral albendazole 400 mg twice per day for 3 days.
- OR single dose of ivermectin 200 µg/kg.

LONG-TERM MANAGEMENT ISSUES

Long-term sequelae are rare. The infestation is ultimately self-limiting since the larva dies after several weeks. Advice should be given about wearing appropriate shoes and beachwear.

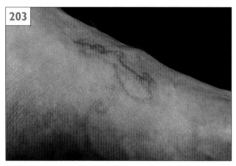

203 Cutaneous larva migrans. A serpiginous track on the dorsum of the foot shows the meanderings of the hookworm larva.

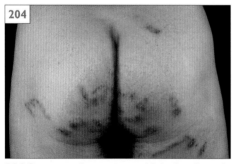

204 Cutaneous larva migrans. Multiple inflamed tracks and nodules on the buttocks. This patient had been sitting on a Caribbean beach contaminated by dog faeces.

Furuncular myiasis

Myiasis is the infestation of body tissues by the larvae of Diptera (two-winged flies). *Dermatobia hominis* (human botfly) is the cause of furuncular myiasis in South America, other species may cause myiasis in North America and Africa. The female botfly deposits her eggs on the abdomen of a vector, such as a mosquito, and these are introduced into the host when the insect takes a blood meal. If undisturbed, larval development within the patient's skin lasts approximately 50–60 days following which the larva emerges, drops to the ground, and pupates.

CLINICAL FEATURES
The initial lesion in furuncular myiasis is a small red papule which is usually seen on the exposed skin of the face, arms, and legs. As the larva grows, the lesion enlarges into a painful, boil-like nodule with a central punctum. The posterior end of the larva, which is equipped with spiracles needed for breathing, is sometimes visible in the punctum (**205**).

DIFFERENTIAL DIAGNOSIS
- Furuncle (p. 120, red, tender abscess arising from a hair follicle).
- Epidermoid cyst (dome-shaped cyst with punctum, may be inflamed).
- Cutaneous leishmaniasis (p. 173, crusted nodule or plaque at site of sandfly bite).

COMPLICATIONS
- Regional lymphadenopathy (with secondary bacterial infection).
- Lymphangitis (with secondary bacterial infection).
- Erysipelas/cellulitis (with secondary bacterial infection).

INVESTIGATIONS
- The diagnosis is made clinically.
- Swab for bacteriology (if secondary infection is suspected).

IMMEDIATE MANAGEMENT
Topical therapy
- Occlusion of the punctum with white soft paraffin ointment will prevent the larva from breathing and provoke it to migrate out.
- Surgical extraction of the larva is also curative.

Systemic therapy
- Treat secondary infection with oral antibiotics.

LONG-TERM MANAGEMENT ISSUES
Resolution of the nodule is usual once the larva has been removed. If the larva is incompletely removed a foreign body reaction may develop.

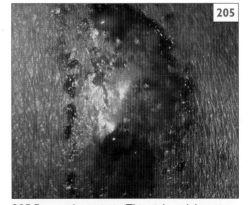

205 Furuncular myiasis. This pink nodule was acquired following a trip to the Amazon and contains the larva of the human botfly. The posterior end of the larva is visible at the upper end of the lesion.

Tungiasis

Tungiasis is a localized inflammation of the skin caused by infestation with the female sand-flea, *Tunga penetrans*, commonly known as the jigger. The jigger flea is common in Africa and Central and South America. The pregnant female flea burrows into the skin of the feet. Once embedded, the flea's eggs develop and enlarge her abdomen to the size of a pea. Subsequently the eggs are released over a 2-week period, after which the female flea dies.

CLINICAL FEATURES

Common sites for a jigger are between the toes, on the soles, or under the toenails. Initially, all that may be visible is a small black dot which is intensely itchy. Later a pale nodule with a dark centre develops (**206, 207**). Examination with a dermatoscope demonstrates pulsations of the embedded female flea. Secondary skin infection is common.

DIFFERENTIAL DIAGNOSIS

- Viral wart (solitary or multiple hyperkeratotic papules or nodules).
- Eccrine poroma (warty nodule with surrounding moat on side of foot or toe).
- Furuncular myiasis (p. 171, painful nodule containing fly larva).

COMPLICATIONS

- Lymphangitis (with secondary bacterial infection).
- Erysipelas/cellulitis (with secondary bacterial infection).
- Tetanus (with secondary infection).

INVESTIGATIONS

- The diagnosis is made clinically.
- Skin swab for bacteriology (if secondary infection is suspected).

IMMEDIATE MANAGEMENT
Topical therapy

- Remove the jigger surgically via curettage.

Systemic therapy

- Give oral antibiotics if secondary infection is present.
- Give tetanus booster, if necessary.

LONG-TERM MANAGEMENT ISSUES

Travellers to tropical countries should be aware of the condition and should be advised to wear appropriate footwear.

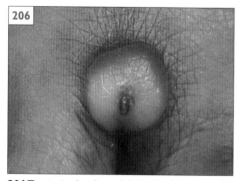

206 Tungiasis. A pale nodule in the first toe web. The flea is visible in the centre of the lesion. This jigger was acquired in Tanzania.

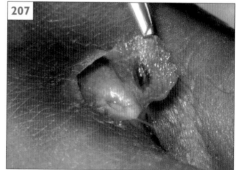

207 Tungiasis. Same patient as in **206**. Lifting the roof of the lesion reveals the female jigger flea embedded in the skin.

Leishmaniasis

Leishmaniasis is a protozoal disease with a wide spectrum of clinical manifestations, including cutaneous and visceral forms. It is caused by species of the genus *Leishmania* transmitted through the bite of the sandfly. Old World leishmaniasis occurs in the countries of the Mediterranean basin (southern Europe, north Africa, Middle East) – the responsible species are: *L. major*, *L. tropica*, *L. aethiopica*, *L. donovani*, and *L. donovani infantum*. New World leishmaniasis occurs in Central and South America – the responsible species include *L. mexicana mexicana*, *L. mexicana amazonensis*, and *L. brasiliensis* complex.

CLINICAL FEATURES

After an incubation period ranging from a few days to several months, one or more lesions appear on exposed skin, particularly the face, neck, and arms. The initial lesion is a nodule which develops a crusted surface and expands over several weeks, reaching a diameter of 3–6 cm (**208**). The crust may fall away to expose a painless ulcer with a raised margin (**209**). Healing generally occurs over the following 6 months, leaving a scar. Disseminated cutaneous leishmaniasis can occur, particularly with infection by *L. aethiopica*. In this form there is extensive spread from the initial lesion with the development of numerous, secondary, nonulcerating nodules. *L. donovani donovani* and *L. donovani infantum* can cause visceral disease (see below).

DIFFERENTIAL DIAGNOSIS

- Atypical mycobacterial infection (violaceous nodule or plaque at site of inoculation of *Mycobacterium marinum* or *M. kansasii*).
- Furuncular myiasis (p. 171, painful nodule containing fly larva).
- Keratoacanthoma (p. 188, firm nodule with keratin plug).
- Tropical ulcer (ulcer on foot or lower leg caused by infection by two or more organisms).
- Cat-scratch disease (crusted papule at site of *Bartonella henselae* inoculation plus regional lymphadenopathy).

COMPLICATIONS

- Regional lymphadenopathy.
- Mucocutaneous leishmaniasis.
- Visceral leishmaniasis:
  - Cough.
  - Diarrhoea.
  - Splenomegaly (can be marked).
  - Hepatomegaly.

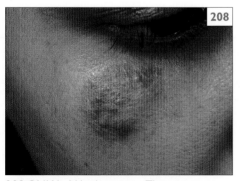

208 Old World leishmaniasis. There is an inflamed red plaque on the cheek of a patient who had travelled to Algeria 3 months earlier.

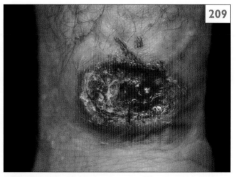

209 Old World leishmaniasis. There is a large ulcerated lesion with indurated margins on the wrist. This patient had been bitten by sandflies in Iran.

INVESTIGATIONS

- Giemsa-stained fine needle aspirate taken from ulcer edge (microscopy reveals amastigotes).
- Skin biopsy for histopathology (mixed dermal infiltrate of macrophages and lymphocytes; amastigotes (Leishman–Donovan bodies) within the cytoplasm of the macrophages).
- Skin biopsy for PCR and culture (specific PCR primers will yield a rapid result; *Leishmania* take up to 10 days to culture in Novy–MacNeal–Nicolle (NNN) medium).

IMMEDIATE MANAGEMENT

New World leishmaniasis should be treated systemically (see below) since the potential for mucocutaneous disease is high. Local treatments can be used for Old World leishmaniasis.

Topical therapy

- Single lesions can be left to heal spontaneously.
- For isolated lesions, local destructive therapies can be used, e.g. surgery or cryotherapy.

Systemic therapy

- For severe infections, systemic sodium stibogluconate (20 mg antimony/kg) for 15–21 days. Diffuse cutaneous leishmaniasis requires systemic antimonial therapy continued for several months after clinical and parasitic clearance.
- Itraconazole also appears to be effective in some cases.

LONG-TERM MANAGEMENT ISSUES

Up to 40% of patients infected with *L. brasiliensis* complex may develop mucocutaneous disease after months to years. Mucosal lesions can result in perforation of the nasal, palatal, and laryngeal cartilages. Post-kala-azar leishmaniasis is a sequel to treated or resolved visceral disease. Clinically there is a papular rash or hypopigmented macules: the papular form tends to resolve spontaneously, whereas the hypopigmented form often persists and becomes nodular. Prevention of leishmaniasis is based on the use of insect repellents and the management of sandfly numbers and activity.

Onchocerciasis

Onchocerciasis (river blindness) is an infection by the filiarial parasite *Onchocerca volvulus*. The infestation mainly involves the skin and eyes. Onchocerciasis occurs predominantly in tropical Africa, but is also encountered in Central and South America. It is transmitted by the black fly (genus *Simulium*) which is found mainly by rivers, hence 'river blindness'. Infected larvae are transmitted via the black fly directly into human skin where they mature into adult worms in subcutaneous tissues. The adult worms produce microfilariae which migrate to the dermis and eye and invade lymphatics. Within the skin, dead and degenerating microfilariae induce an inflammatory reaction which results in a range of cutaneous syndromes including an acute and highly symptomatic dermatosis.

CLINICAL FEATURES

Acute papular onchodermatitis is characterized by numerous small papules or pustules mainly on the shoulders, buttocks, and hips which are intensely itchy. The eruption may be urticarial or oedematous. In Central America, itchy facial swelling is also a manifestation of acute disease. In chronic onchodermatitis there are excoriated papules, generalized lichenification, hyperpigmentation, and coarse wrinkles, particularly of the torso and buttocks (**210**). Marked axillary and inguinal lymphadenopathy is typical with chronic involvement. Depigmentation with perifollicular pigment retention is a late feature of onchocerciasis. Subcutaneous nodules are often present over bony prominences.

DIFFERENTIAL DIAGNOSIS
Acute papular onchodermatitis

- Atopic dermatitis (p. 18, eczema on face, torso, and flexures as part of atopic diathesis).
- Scabies infestation (p. 162, severe pruritus plus burrows at the wrists and finger webs).

Chronic onchodermatitis

- Nodular prurigo (lichenified nodules on torso and limbs from persistent scratching).
- Chronic eczema (lichenification, scaling, depigmentation, and coarse wrinkling).
- Leprosy (lepromatous – thickened skin, leonine facies; tuberculoid – hypopigmented patches).

COMPLICATIONS

- Conjunctivitis.
- Sclerosing keratitis.
- Uveitis.
- Optic atrophy.
- Glaucoma.
- Blindness.
- Regional lymphadenopathy.
- Lymphoedema (especially genital).

INVESTIGATIONS

- Diagnosis is often clinical in endemic areas.
- Skin snip microscopy (examination of skin sample immersed in saline should demonstrate emerging microfilariae within 1–4 hr).
- Filarial immunofluorescence test or enzyme-linked immunosorbent assay (ELISA) (positive in 60–90% cases).
- Blood count (eosinophilia).
- Skin biopsy for histopathology (dermal inflammatory cell infiltrate including eosinophils with microfilariae between collagen bundles).

IMMEDIATE MANAGEMENT
Systemic therapy

- One dose of ivermectin 100–200 µg/kg is given. A second treatment may be needed after 6–12 months.

LONG-TERM MANAGEMENT ISSUES

The major complication of onchocerciasis is visual impairment; it is the commonest cause of blindness in endemic areas. Prevention of onchocerciasis is based on the use of insect repellents and the management of black fly numbers and activity.

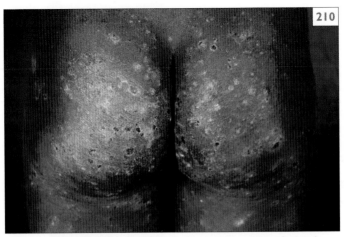

210 Chronic onchodermatitis. There are numerous lichenified and excoriated nodules on the buttocks of this patient from the Congo.

Sporotrichosis

Skin infection by the fungus *Sporothrix schenkii* causes sporotrichosis which can present both as an acute and chronic dermatosis. Systemic sporotrichosis also occurs, particularly in immunosuppressed individuals. *S. schenkii* grows on rotten wood and other decaying vegetable matter and is found in temperate zones (USA, Canada) and tropical climates (Central and South America, Africa). In cutaneous sporotrichosis the fungus is introduced into the skin through a minor wound (often via injury from a rose thorn), while in systemic sporotrichosis transmission is via inhalation. The incubation period ranges from 8–30 days.

CLINICAL FEATURES

Two forms of cutaneous sporotrichosis occur; lymphangitic type and fixed type. Infection occurs when the fungus is implanted at the site of injury, usually on exposed sites such as arms and hands. The lymphangitic form presents as a painless nodule or pustule which develops several weeks after the injury. Subsequently the nodule ulcerates and discharges. Thereafter secondary nodules develop over the draining lymphatics, spreading proximally in a 'sporotrichoid' pattern (**211**). In the fixed form there is a solitary ulcerating nodule or verrucous lesion. In systemic sporotrichosis pulmonary involvement is usual and occurs preferentially in patients with chronic obstructive pulmonary disease or alcoholism.

DIFFERENTIAL DIAGNOSIS

- Atypical mycobacterial infection (violaceous nodule or plaque at site of inoculation of *M. marinum* or *M. kansasii*, shows sporotrichoid spread).
- Cutaneous leishmaniasis (p. 173, crusted nodule or plaque at site of sandfly bite).
- Cat-scratch disease (crusted papule at site of *Bartonella henselae* inoculation plus regional lymphadenopathy).

COMPLICATIONS

- Regional lymphadenopathy.
- Pulmonary sporotrichosis.

INVESTIGATIONS

- Skin biopsy for histopathology (granulomatous and suppurative inflammation in dermis; asteroid bodies; organisms are often not seen).
- Skin biopsy for culture (microscopic examination of cultured organism reveals diagnostic features).

IMMEDIATE MANAGEMENT
Systemic therapy

- Oral itraconazole 100 mg once daily for 3 months.
- Amphotericin B in severe or disseminated disease.

LONG-TERM MANAGEMENT ISSUES

At-risk individuals (e.g. gardeners) should be aware of the condition and should be advised to wear appropriate gloves and hand protection.

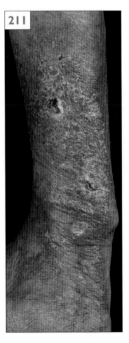

211 Sporotrichosis. These inflamed lesions developed proximally (sporotrichoid spread) over the wrist and forearm following an injury to the hand. The most proximal nodule has ulcerated.

Rickettsial spotted fevers

The Rickettsiae are Gram-negative micro-organisms which cause 'spotted' fevers, the most important being Rocky Mountain spotted fever (*Rickettsia rickettsii*) and Mediterranean spotted fever (*Rickettsia conorii*). Rocky Mountain spotted fever occurs in eastern USA and Brazil. Mediterranean spotted fever (MSF) is found around the Mediterranean, especially in Israel. Rickettsiae are transmitted to humans by the bite of infected arthropod vectors, usually ticks. Seasonal variation in the prevalence of spotted fevers reflects tick numbers; the majority of cases occur during the summer months when tick activity is high. If untreated the rickettsial spotted fevers are associated with significant morbidity and mortality.

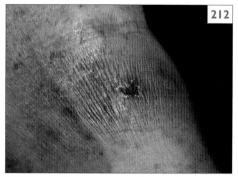

212 Rocky Mountain spotted fever. An eschar (known as the 'tache noire') develops at the site of the tick bite prior to the widespread eruption of a rickettsial spotted fever, in this case Rocky Mountain spotted fever.

CLINICAL FEATURES

There are four main features which occur during a rickettsial spotted fever: (1) an inoculation eschar ('tache noire') at the site of the tick bite (**212**); (2) a maculo-papular or purpuric eruption (**213**); (3) lymphadenopathy; (4) fever. In Rocky Mountain spotted fever, a high fever and constitutional symptoms develop 6–8 days after the tick bite; 2–4 days later a red, macular eruption appears, initially localized to the wrists and ankles. Subsequently the rash becomes maculo-papular, petechial, and generalized, involving the palms and soles but sparing the face (**214**). In severe cases the lesions can be purpuric. A wide range of systemic features can accompany the rash and mortality can be as high as 25% in untreated cases, or higher in the elderly.

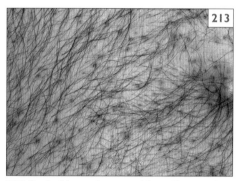

213 Rocky Mountain spotted fever. Same patient as in **212**. An exanthem of tiny petechial macules on the torso is typical. The patient also had a fever, myalgia, and lymphadenopathy.

DIFFERENTIAL DIAGNOSIS

- Viral exanthem (p. 140, a widespread morbilliform eruption with flu-like symptoms).
- Drug-induced exanthem (p. 220, a morbilliform eruption on torso and limbs).
- Small vessel vasculitis (p. 82, palpable purpura on dependent areas).
- Meningococcal septicaemia (p. 130, localized or widespread purpura).
- Dengue fever (p. 178, morbilliform eruption or confluent erythema with islands of sparing).

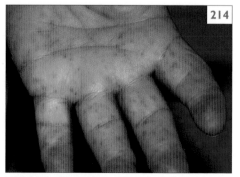

214 Rocky Mountain spotted fever. Same patient as in **212**. Involvement of the palms and soles is typical in rickettsial spotted fevers.

COMPLICATIONS
Complications of Rocky Mountain spotted fever
- Fever (>39°C).
- Headache, malaise.
- Lymphadenopathy.
- Nausea, vomiting.
- Anorexia, diarrhoea.
- Hepatomegaly.
- Abdominal pain, myalgia.
- Seizures, meningitis.
- Dyspnoea, pleural effusions.
- Multiple organ failure.

INVESTIGATIONS
- Blood count (thrombocytopenia).
- Basic chemistry, liver function tests (hyponatraemia, raised transaminases).
- CPK (raised).
- ESR, CRP (raised CRP).
- Clotting studies (prolonged PT and APTT may occur).
- Rickettsial serology: serological studies on paired acute and convalescent sera (serological evidence of infection by 2nd week of illness).

IMMEDIATE MANAGEMENT
Systemic therapy
- Doxycycline 100 mg (oral or IV) is given twice daily for 7 days (it should be continued for 3 days after resolution of fever).

Supportive therapy
- The patient must be admitted to hospital for monitoring of vital signs, administration of therapy (see above), and management of complications.

LONG-TERM MANAGEMENT ISSUES
Prevention of rickettsial spotted fevers is based on the avoidance of ticks using chemical repellents and protective clothing. Report any case of a rickettsial spotted fever to the public health authorities.

Dengue

Dengue is caused by infection with one of the dengue viruses which are transmitted to humans by *Aedes* mosquito bites. Infection causes a range of disorders, notably dengue fever, dengue haemorrhagic fever, and dengue shock syndrome. Dengue is widespread in tropical and subtropical areas of Africa, Central and South America, Oceania and Southeast Asia. Localized epidemics occur frequently in affected countries and it is not uncommon for travellers to these areas to become infected. However, dengue is unlikely if symptoms appear more than 2 weeks after leaving an endemic area and if the fever lasts longer than 10 days.

CLINICAL FEATURES
Dengue fever starts after an incubation period of 4–7 days and tends to be a self-limiting illness which lasts 7–10 days. Early on in dengue fever patients develop fever, headache, nausea, and vomiting. Facial flushing is a common feature and musculoskeletal symptoms are prominent. The rash of dengue fever occurs in approximately 50% of patients and appears on the 3rd day of the fever. It is characterized by a morbilliform exanthem or confluent erythema containing zones of unaffected skin (islands of sparing) (**215–217**). The rash fades as the fever subsides at around day 7. Dengue haemorrhagic fever is more common in children and is characterized by the same set of features accompanied by a haemorrhagic diathesis with petechiae, purpura, mucosal bleeding, and bleeding from venepuncture sites. In some patients dengue haemorrhagic fever can proceed to shock (dengue shock syndrome) which carries a high mortality rate.

DIFFERENTIAL DIAGNOSIS
- Viral exanthem (p. 140, a widespread morbilliform eruption with flu-like symptoms).
- Drug-induced exanthem (p. 220, a morbilliform eruption on torso and limbs).
- Small vessel vasculitis (p. 82, palpable purpura on dependent areas).
- Meningococcal septicaemia (p. 130, localized or widespread purpura).
- Rickettsial spotted fevers (p. 178, maculo-papular and petechial eruption with eschar from tick bite).

- Other viral haemorrhagic fevers, e.g. Ebola, Marburg (morbilliform exanthem with fever, headache, myalgia, hepatitis, renal damage, and haemorrhage).

COMPLICATIONS
- Fever and prostration.
- Headache.
- Nausea and vomiting.
- Joint and bone pain ('break bone fever').
- Myalgia causing severe back pain.

INVESTIGATIONS
- Blood count (leucopenia with lymphocytopenia occurs at the end of the febrile illness; a raised haematocrit is associated with the haemorrhagic tendency; thrombocytopenia accompanies dengue haemorrhagic fever and dengue shock syndrome).
- Basic chemistry, liver function tests (hyponatraemia and a mild rise in transaminases).
- Clotting studies (prolonged PT and APTT occur in dengue haemorrhagic fever).
- ESR, CRP (raised CRP).
- Serum: PCR of virus, culture of virus.
- Serum: serological studies on paired acute and convalescent sera.

IMMEDIATE MANAGEMENT
Systemic therapy
There is no specific therapy for Dengue.
- Paracetamol (acetaminophen) for fever.
- Opiate analgesia may be required.

Supportive therapy
- The patient must be admitted to hospital for monitoring of vital signs, administration of intravenous fluids, and management of complications.
- Patients with dengue shock syndrome need to be managed on an ITU.

LONG-TERM MANAGEMENT ISSUES
Complete recovery from dengue fever is usual, whereas the mortality rate from dengue shock syndrome is 10–40%. Infection with one dengue serotype confers lifelong immunity, however at-risk individuals can eventually be infected by all four dengue viruses. In order to limit infection vector avoidance is important (clothing, insect repellent). Report any case of dengue infection to the public health authorities.

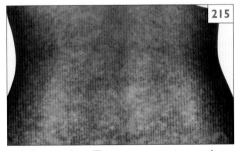

215 Dengue fever. There is a purpuric exanthem on this patient with dengue who had recently returned from travelling in Southeast Asia. She also had a fever, severe bone pain, and myalgia.

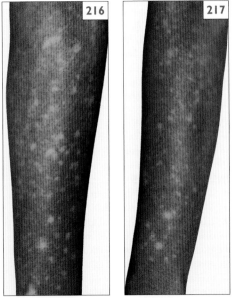

216, 217 Dengue fever. Same patient as in **215**. There are islands of sparing within the exanthem. This is typical for dengue.

Swimmer's itch

Swimmer's itch or cercarial dermatitis is a form of cutaneous schistosomiasis which occurs after swimming in freshwater infested with cercaria of avian schistosomes. Schistosomiasis is endemic in many countries of the tropics and subtropics and the risk of infection is highest during the summer when cercariae are most numerous.

CLINICAL FEATURES
Swimmer's itch occurs within hours of contact with infected water. There is an itchy eruption on exposed sites. Red macules appear initially which develop into small pruritic papules (**218**). The lesions tend to persist for 5–7 days before resolving spontaneously.

DIFFERENTIAL DIAGNOSIS
- Insect bites (p. 164, itchy, grouped papules with central punctum).
- Sea-bather's eruption (p. 181, small, itchy red papules on sites covered by swimwear).

COMPLICATIONS
- Katayama fever (systemic allergic reaction during acute phase of infection).

INVESTIGATIONS
- The diagnosis is usually made clinically.
- Blood count (eosinophilia).
- ELISA for schistosomal antibodies (able to distinguish acute from chronic infection).
- Skin biopsy for histopathology (spongiosis and dermal oedema with a mixed inflammatory infiltrate of histiocytes, lymphocytes, and eosinophils).

IMMEDIATE MANAGEMENT
Topical therapy
- Corticosteroid ointment, twice per day (use for restricted period):
    trunk and limbs: potent.

Systemic therapy
- H_1-antihistamine (e.g. levocetirizine 5 mg once daily).

LONG-TERM MANAGEMENT ISSUES
Swimmer's itch can progress to systemic schistosomiasis. For suspected systemic schistosomiasis, give praziquantel as two oral doses of 20 mg/kg on a single day. Bilharziasis cutanea tarda is a chronic dermatosis secondary to the deposition of ova within cutaneous vasculature and is characterized by papular, granulomatous lesions of the anogenital skin. Written and pictorial warnings should be present at lakes known to be infested.

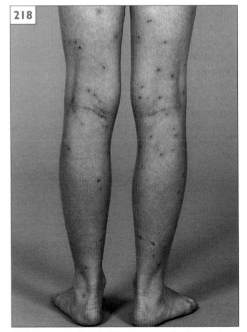

218 Swimmer's itch. There are multiple papules on this girl's legs which appeared within 2 hr of swimming in a lake infected with schistosomiasis.

Sea-bathers' eruption

Sea-bathers' eruption is a dermatosis caused by the stings of jellyfish larvae (*Linuche unguiculata*, known as thimble jellyfish). The eruption occurs on parts of the body covered by the bathing trunks or swimming costume since the larvae, which are the size of a pinhead, pass through the weave of swimwear and become trapped against the skin. Pressure changes trigger the larva's stinging mechanism to inject venom into the skin, which is both toxic and antigenic. Sea-bathers' eruption occurs following bathing in tropical and subtropical coastal waters especially off the eastern coast of Florida, in the Pacific Ocean, and the Caribbean.

CLINICAL FEATURES

Patients report a history of skin 'prickling' which occurs while they are swimming or within a few hours of leaving the water. The rash appears within 4–24 hr following exposure and is characterized by multiple, small, itchy red papules found predominantly on sites covered by swimwear (**219**) or in the flexures. Pustules and vesicles may develop. The lesions heal with crusting over 7–10 days.

DIFFERENTIAL DIAGNOSIS

- Contact dermatitis (p. 18, eczema which is localized or in an unusual distribution).
- Folliculitis (p. 120, follicular papules and pustules).
- Swimmer's itch (p. 180, itchy eruption on exposed sites on swimming in infested freshwater).

COMPLICATIONS

- Fatigue and malaise.
- Headache and nausea.
- Fever.
- Regional lymphadenopathy.

INVESTIGATIONS

The diagnosis is made clinically.

IMMEDIATE MANAGEMENT

Take off swimwear immediately and rinse the skin in noninfested seawater.

Topical therapy

- Corticosteroid ointment, twice per day (use for restricted period):
  trunk and limbs: potent.

Systemic therapy

- NSAIDs may help the symptoms (e.g. naproxen 500 mg twice per day).
- For a severe reaction, a short course of oral corticosteroids can be helpful (e.g. prednisolone 20–30 mg daily for 5 days and reduce by 5 mg every 5th day).

LONG-TERM MANAGEMENT ISSUES

The episode usually settles with symptomatic treatment as outlined above. Recurrent episodes may occur on repeated exposure. Written and pictorial warnings should be present on beaches during outbreaks.

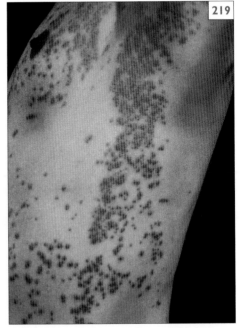

219 Sea-bathers' eruption. This woman had been swimming off the coast of Mexico.

Jellyfish stings

Jellyfish tentacles are covered by hundreds of stinging organs, called nematocysts, which become activated when in contact with skin. A barbed thread is discharged from the nematocyst and inoculates toxin into the victim. Jellyfish which most commonly sting swimmers are called the sea-nettles and are found in the Atlantic, Indian, and Pacific oceans. The Portugese man-of-war, found in both the Atlantic Ocean and Mediterranean Sea, can cause a severe systemic illness as well as a local reaction.

CLINICAL FEATURES

Most jellyfish stings present with an immediate and severe localized, burning pain which persists for up to 1 hr. A red, linear, urticated lesion will develop at the site of the sting (**220**). Due to the distribution of nematocysts a beaded pattern of small weals is often seen. More serious stings cause blisters with erosions or areas of haemorrhagic necrosis. A severe systemic reaction (see below) may occur within 15 minutes of a sting from the box jellyfish or Portugese man-of-war.

DIFFERENTIAL DIAGNOSIS

- Sea anemone dermatitis (local inflammation at site of toxin inoculation from certain species).
- Fire coral sting (painful papulo-pustular eruption following contact with coral).
- Contact dermatitis (p. 18, eczema which is localized or in an unusual distribution).

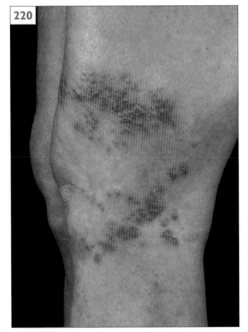

220 Jellyfish sting. The shape of the inflammation conforms to the site of contact with a jellyfish tentacle. The papules are caused by toxin released from the tentacle's nematocysts.

COMPLICATIONS

With box jellyfish or Portugese man-of-war stings:

- Anaphylaxis
- Cardiovascular: arrhythmias, coronary artery vasospasm, cardiomyopathy.
- Respiratory: laryngeal oedema, bronchospasm, respiratory failure.
- Gastrointestinal: nausea, vomiting, hepatic failure.
- Renal: acute renal failure.
- Neurological: headache, neuropsychiatric disturbance, seizures, coma.
- Musculoskeletal: arthritis, muscle spasm, rhabdomyolysis.
- Thrombophlebitis.
- Secondary bacterial infection.
- Regional lymphadenopathy.

INVESTIGATIONS

- The diagnosis is usually made clinically.
- Blood count, routine chemistry, liver function tests (haemolysis, renal impairment, hepatic impairment).
- CPK (rhabdomyolysis).
- ECG (arrhythmias).
- Skin biopsy for histopathology (not usually indicated) (spongiosis of epidermis, red cell extravasation, and an eosinophil-rich mixed inflammatory cell infiltrate; in chronic cases – granulomatous inflammation).
- Confirmation of envenomation and identification of the species can be achieved by tape stripping of nematocysts from the skin.

IMMEDIATE MANAGEMENT
Topical therapy

- Remove any retained nematocysts.
- For suspected box jellyfish stings douse wound with diluted vinegar.
- For suspected sea-nettle stings apply a paste of sodium bicarbonate.
- Corticosteroid ointment, twice per day (use for restricted period):
    trunk and limbs: superpotent.
- If a distal limb has been affected then the use of a gentle tourniquet to cause lymphovenous compression may reduce systemic problems.

Systemic therapy

- Adequate analgesia.
- Specific antivenin can be obtained for certain stings.
- Muscle relaxants for local spasms.
- Oral corticosteroids for severe reactions (e.g. prednisolone 0.5–1 mg/kg once daily).
- Tetanus vaccination, if necessary.
- Systemic antibiotics if secondary infection.

Supportive therapy

With a severe reaction admit to hospital for monitoring of vital signs and administration of therapy (see above).

- Cardiopulmonary resuscitation, if necessary.
- IV fluids, as required.
- Treat anaphylaxis with:
- – IM or SC epinephrine (adrenaline) 0.5–1.0 mg.
- – Slow IV injection of chlorpheniramine 10–20 mg.
- – IV hydrocortisone sodium succinate 100–300 mg.
- – Oxygen.

LONG-TERM MANAGEMENT ISSUES

Cutaneous complications of jellyfish stings include pigmented striae, granulomatous reactions, and keloid scarring. Recurrent episodes of urticaria may occur up to 4 weeks after the event and require symptomatic treatment only. Encourage individuals to swim in patrolled areas only and to wear a wet suit.

Tumours and malignancies

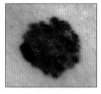 **Malignant melanoma**

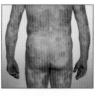 **Mycosis fungoides and Sézary syndrome**

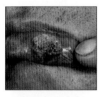 **Squamous cell carcinoma**

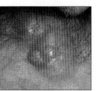 **Primary cutaneous B cell lymphoma**

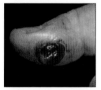 **Pyogenic granuloma**

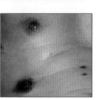 **Cutaneous metastases**

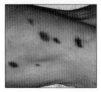 **Kaposi's sarcoma**

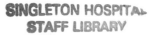

Malignant melanoma

Malignant melanoma (MM) is a tumour of melanocytes, predominantly of the skin. Risk factors for MM include: fair skin (especially with red hair and freckles), a history of excessive exposure to strong sunlight, the presence of numerous melanocytic naevi (particularly clinically atypical moles), and a family history of MM. In most cases MM passes through an initial radial growth phase prior to adopting an invasive and metastasing phenotype (vertical growth phase). Melanomas which are greater than 4 mm in depth at presentation are associated with a mortality rate of 50% at 5 years. All patients with a suspected MM should be referred urgently to a dermatologist.

CLINICAL FEATURES
Any new pigmented lesion appearing on the skin or any pre-existing pigmented lesion undergoing change in size, shape or colour should be considered a MM until proven otherwise. The most significant clinical features are: (1) an increase in diameter, (2) the development of an irregular outline, (3) a variation of the pigmentation within the lesion. Most melanomas can be assigned to one of six clinical sub-types: superficial spreading (**221**), nodular (**222**), acral lentiginous (**223**), subungual (**224**), amelanotic (**225**), and lentigo maligna melanoma (**226**). These categories, which describe morphological or site characteristics, have some bearing on prognosis, for example superficial spreading melanoma has a good prognosis, while nodular melanoma has a poor prognosis. Examination of pigmented lesions can be enhanced by the use of a dermatoscope. The presence of a suspected MM should prompt the examination of regional lymph nodes for lymphadenopathy.

DIFFERENTIAL DIAGNOSIS
- Benign melanocytic naevus (symmetrical lesion with smooth outline and uniform pigment distribution).
- Seborrhoeic keratosis (often pigmented with a roughened, warty surface).
- Spitz naevus (red–brown nodule, usually in children).
- Blue naevus (blue–black papule or nodule).
- Pigmented basal cell carcinoma (nodule or plaque with a translucent margin, surface telangiectasiae, and pigment).
- Pyogenic granuloma (p. 191, fleshy, red or purple nodule, may be mistaken for an amelanotic melanoma).

COMPLICATIONS
Metastatic spread to:
- Lymph nodes.
- Liver.
- Brain.
- Bone.
- Skin.
- Other organs.

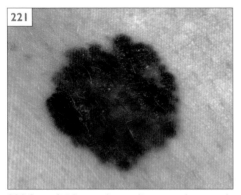

221 Superficial spreading malignant melanoma. A flat, brown lesion which has unevenly distributed pigment and a notched, irregular margin.

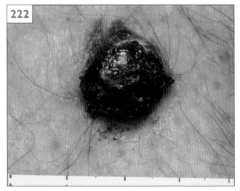

222 Nodular malignant melanoma. A black, ulcerated nodule.

INVESTIGATIONS

- Excise the whole suspected MM plus a margin of clinically normal surrounding skin of at least 2 mm. *The sample must be sent for histopathology.*
- Skin histopathology (a tumour of cytologically malignant melanocytes invading the dermis; the depth of the tumour, Breslow thickness, is the best prognostic guide to 5-year survival; ulceration, atypical mitoses, a lymphocytic infiltrate, and a lack of melanocyte maturation are features which indicate an aggressive behaviour).

- In tumours which have ulcerated and/or have a Breslow thickness greater than 2 mm, perform the following investigations:
- Chest radiography, liver ultrasonography, CT or positron emission tomography (PET) scan of chest, abdomen, and pelvis (if metastatic spread is suspected).
- Blood count, basic chemistry, liver function tests (as indicators of general health and if metastatic spread is suspected).
- LDH (as indicator of tumour burden).

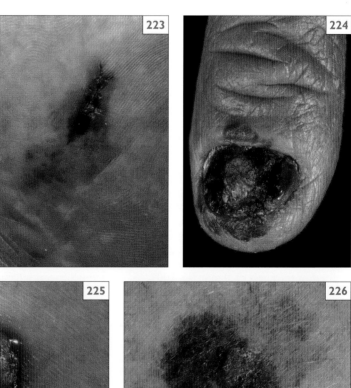

223 Acral lentiginous malignant melanoma. There is a zone of black within a larger area of pale pigmentation on the plantar skin.

224 Subungual malignant melanoma. The melanoma has destroyed the nail plate. Pigment has spread on to the proximal nail fold and the tip of the digit.

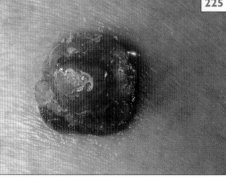

225 Amelanotic malignant melanoma. A pink, fleshy nodule with an ulcerated surface.

226 Lentigo maligna melanoma. There is a thickened area (invasive melanoma) within this irregular pigmented macule (lentigo maligna) on the face.

IMMEDIATE MANAGEMENT

Excise the lesion (see investigations). Since there is no effective treatment for disseminated MM it is imperative that early tumours are recognized promptly and excised without delay.

LONG-TERM MANAGEMENT ISSUES

Breslow thickness of the MM should guide subsequent local excision of the primary wound: in a tumour with a Breslow thickness of 0.1–1 mm, excise the wound with a 1 cm margin; with a Breslow thickness of 1–2 mm, excise with a 1–2 cm margin; with a Breslow thickness of >2 mm excise with a 2–3 cm margin. Patients may be considered for sentinel lymph node biopsy if the Breslow thickness is >1 mm and <4 mm. Localized lymph node involvement can be treated with lymph node dissection. Loco-regional recurrent melanoma may be treated with infusion of cytotoxic agent or CO_2 ablation of superficial lesions. For widely disseminated metastatic disease, high-dose interferon-α or chemotherapy with dacarbazine can be offered. Patients who have had a MM should practice careful photo-protection and receive regular follow-up by a dermatologist. Follow-up consultations should include an examination for local, regional or distant metastasis and a full skin check to exclude the development of a further primary melanoma. The management of MM requires the expertise of a multidisciplinary team including dermatologists, plastic surgeons, oncologists, specialist nurses, and pathologists.

The five-year survival rates are as follows:
- Breslow thickness <1.0 mm: 95–100%.
- Breslow thickness 1–2.0 mm: 80–95%.
- Breslow thickness 2.1–4.0 mm: 60–75%.
- Breslow thickness >4.0 mm: 50%.

Squamous cell carcinoma

Squamous cell carcinoma (SCC) is a malignant tumour arising from keratinocytes in the epidermis and stratified squamous mucosa. It is locally invasive and has the potential to metastasize. SCCs occur most commonly in fair-skinned individuals who have received a high cumulative exposure to strong sunlight. Patients taking immunosuppresive medication (e.g. solid organ transplant recipients) also have a greater risk of developing cutaneous SCC. All patients with a suspected SCC should be referred urgently to a dermatologist.

CLINICAL FEATURES

SCC usually arises on sun-exposed sites in individuals aged 50 years and above. The surrounding skin often shows evidence of solar damage (freckling, dryness, solar keratoses). An SCC may develop within a patch of Bowen's disease (intraepidermal SCC) or arise at a chronic scar or ulcer (Marjolin's ulcer). Most commonly affected sites are the helix of the ear, the nose, the lower lip (**227**), and the dorsal aspect of the hands and forearms (**228**). The tumour is usually a nodule but may present as a papule, plaque, or ulcer (**227–232**). SCCs can be painful and on palpation are often firm and indurated. Well differentiated SCCs show evidence of keratinization with scaling or horn formation, while poorly differentiated lesions are fleshy and friable. The surface may become eroded or crusted and show signs of secondary staphylococcal infection. A keratoacanthoma (KA) is a well differentiated, low-grade SCC which has the capacity to undergo self-healing. Clinically a KA is a skin-coloured, dome-shaped nodule with a central keratin plug (**232**). KAs tend to grow rapidly to 1–2 cm in diameter. The presence of a suspected SCC should prompt the examination of regional lymph nodes for lymphadenopathy.

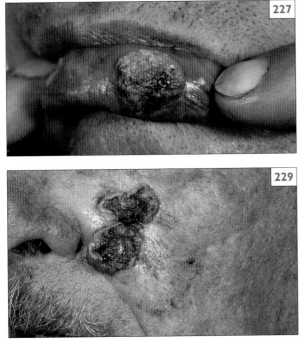

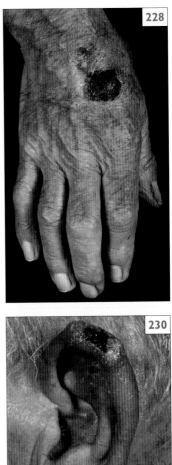

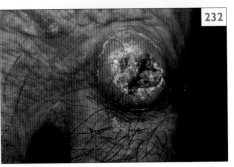

227 Squamous cell carcinoma. The lower lip is a common site for SCC in smokers.

228 Squamous cell carcinoma. This man with an SCC on the back of his hand gave a history of excessive sun exposure.

229 Squamous cell carcinoma. A large ulcerated plaque with rolled edges on the face of a man with other features of photodamage.

230 Squamous cell carcinoma. This ulcerated SCC on the pinna had metastasized to regional lymph nodes.

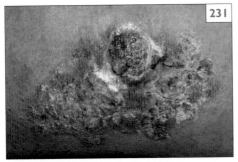

231 Squamous cell carcinoma. A fleshy nodule (SCC) arising within a patch of Bowen's disease (SCC *in situ*).

232 Keratoacanthoma. Typically a KA is a round, dome-shaped nodule with a central keratin plug.

DIFFERENTIAL DIAGNOSIS
- Basal cell carcinoma (nodule or plaque with telangiectasiae and a translucent margin; may ulcerate).
- Viral wart (skin-coloured papule or nodule with warty surface, sometimes peduculated).
- Amelanotic melanoma (p. 186, red, fleshy nodule, often with a moist eroded surface).
- Chondrodermatitis nodularis helicis (firm, tender nodule on the helix of the ear).

COMPLICATIONS
Metastatic spread to:
- Lymph nodes.
- Lungs.
- Liver.
- Other organs.

INVESTIGATIONS
- Instead of taking a diagnostic biopsy it is preferable to excise the whole suspected SCC plus a margin of clinically normal surrounding skin of at least 2 mm. *The sample must be sent for histopathology.*
- Skin histopathology (nests of pleomorphic squamous cells arising from the epidermis and invading the dermis; the cells have eosinophilic cytoplasm and vesicular nuclei; there is variable keratinization depending on the degree of tumour differentiation).

IMMEDIATE TREATMENT
Surgical excision of the SCC with a margin of surrounding normal skin is the optimal treatment. A 4 mm margin is appropriate for well defined tumours which are <2 cm in diameter. High-risk tumours (>2 cm in diameter and 4 mm in depth; poorly differentiated; immunosuppressed patient; situated on lip or ear) should be removed with a 6 mm margin. Where there is difficulty in determining the surgical border or at sites where tissue conservation is important, microscopically guided surgery is recommended (Mohs micrographic surgery).

Local destruction with curettage and cautery may be used in patients with extensive actinic damage and multiple SCCs which are <1 cm in diameter. However, curettage is associated with a higher risk of recurrence. In elderly patients who are unable to tolerate surgery, radiotherapy is an alternative treatment modality.

LONG-TERM MANAGEMENT ISSUES
The management of SCC requires the expertise of a multidisciplinary team including dermatologists, plastic surgeons, oncologists, specialist nurses, and pathologists. Local recurrence and metastasis of an SCC is dependent on the following features: being greater than 2 cm in diameter and 4 mm in depth; being poorly differentiated; arising in patients who are immunosuppressed; occurring at high-risk sites (e.g. lip, ear). All patients who have had an SCC should practice careful photoprotection and receive regular follow-up by a dermatologist who should examine for: signs of recurrence, regional or distant metastasis, and new lesions. Recipients of an organ transplant should also undergo regular skin surveillance for early detection and treatment of SCC. Long-term systemic retinoid therapy can reduce the development of new squamoproliferative lesions in individuals with a history of multiple SCCs.

Pyogenic granuloma

A pyogenic granuloma is a vascular nodule (benign capillary haemangioma) which grows rapidly, often following minor skin trauma. Pyogenic granulomas have a tendency to bleed causing patients to seek an urgent opinion. There is an association with pregnancy.

CLINICAL FEATURES

A pyogenic granuloma is most commonly situated on a finger or a lip. The lesion is a dark red nodule measuring 0.5–2.0 cm in diameter (**233, 234**). The base may be pedunculated, the surface is often eroded and sometimes covered by impetiginized crust. Pyogenic granulomas are usually painless but tend to bleed when knocked.

DIFFERENTIAL DIAGNOSIS

- Amelanotic melanoma (p. 186, red, fleshy nodule, often with a moist eroded surface).
- Other haemangiomas (smooth-surfaced red–purple papule or nodule).
- Viral wart (skin-coloured papule with warty surface, sometimes peduculated).
- Keratoacanthoma (p. 188, skin-coloured, dome-shaped nodule with a central keratin plug).
- Inflamed seborrhoeic wart (often pigmented with a roughened, warty surface).

COMPLICATIONS

There usually none.

- Rarely anaemia (with chronic, persistent bleeding).

INVESTIGATIONS

- The lesions should be excised and sent for histopathology.
- Skin histopathology (a lobular proliferation of small blood vessels which often breaches the epidermis producing an ulcerated pedunculated tumour).

IMMEDIATE MANAGEMENT

Excision or curettage and cautery are carried out under local anaesthetic. It is important to remove a section of skin under the lesion by excision or deep curettage since any retained proliferating vessels in the dermis may result in recurrence of the pyogenic granuloma.

LONG-TERM MANAGEMENT ISSUES

A proportion of pyogenic granulomas will recur following surgical removal and necessitate further, more aggressive surgical intervention.

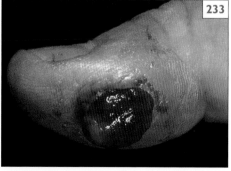

233 Pyogenic granuloma. There is a red, friable nodule on the finger with signs of recent bleeding. Fingers are a common site for a pyogenic granuloma.

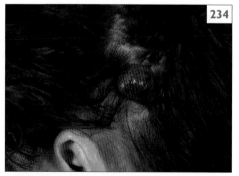

234 Pyogenic granuloma. There is a large, dark red, pedunculated tumour on the scalp.

Kaposi's sarcoma

Kaposi's sarcoma (KS) usually presents on the skin but is a systemic, multifocal disease. There are four clinical sub-types: (1) classic KS which affects elderly men from southern Europe or Jews of eastern European descent; (2) African endemic KS which occurs in equatorial Africa and again affects men predominantly; (3) KS in iatrogenically immunocompromised patients, usually organ transplant recipients; (4) HIV-related KS. All types are associated with human herpesvirus (HHV) type 8 infection (HHV8). Although KS runs a chronic course many cases are associated with serious immunosuppression and therefore prompt diagnosis is essential.

CLINICAL FEATURES

KS lesions are purple in colour. Lesions may begin as macular patches, especially in iatrogenic KS, but progress to become well defined papules or nodules, often multiple (235, 236). Lesions may coalesce and ulcerate. All sites, including mucosal surfaces, can be involved but lesions are most frequently seen on the legs (237). The disease can progress to affect lymph nodes and internal organs, with lung involvement having a particularly poor prognosis. The clinical course is variable; rapid spread can occur in endemic KS and HIV-related KS, whereas classic KS typically has a slow progression. KS involvement of lymphatics can cause lymphoedema.

DIFFERENTIAL DIAGNOSIS

- Other haemangiomas (smooth-surfaced red–purple papule or nodule).
- Cutaneous metastasis (p. 198, painless red–blue or red–brown nodule).
- Amelanotic melanoma (p. 186, red, fleshy nodule, often with a moist eroded surface).
- B cell lymphoma (p. 196, red or red–brown nodule or plaque).
- Acroangiodermatitis of venous insufficiency (purple patches or plaques on lower legs).
- Bacillary angiomatosis (angioproliferative disease caused by *Bartonella* infection in immunocompromised individuals).

COMPLICATIONS

- Organ involvement with associated haemorrhage (small bowel and lung).
- Lymphadenopathy.
- Lymphoedema.

INVESTIGATIONS

- Blood count and T cell subsets (lymphopenia in immunosuppression, low CD4 count in HIV infection).
- HIV test.
- Skin biopsy for histopathology (dermal proliferation of small vessels and slit-like spaces separating collagen bundles with sparse lymphoplasmacytic infiltrate; spindle cells express vascular markers (e.g. CD31); vascular channels contain erythrocytes).
- Staging investigations: chest radiography, ultrasonography of liver, CT scan of chest, abdomen, and pelvis.

IMMEDIATE MANAGEMENT

In immunodeficient patients, the cause of immunosuppression should be addressed where possible. This may include adjusting immunosuppressive therapy in organ recipients or starting highly active antiretroviral therapy in HIV infection.

LONG-TERM MANAGEMENT ISSUES

The management of KS requires the expertise of a multidisciplinary team, including dermatologists, pathologists, oncologists, radiotherapists, specialist nurses, and, where appropriate, HIV physicians. Single lesions may be treated by surgery, cryotherapy, or intralesional chemotherapy (vinblastine). Radiotherapy is the treatment of choice for localized KS. Chemotherapy may be required for rapidly progressing or widespread systemic disease: agents used either singularly or in combination include vincristine, chlorambucil, cyclophosphamide, doxorubicin, daunorubicin, and paclitaxel. Other treatments include interferon-α and gemcitabine. In older immunocompetent patients with indolent disease, observation alone may be appropriate.

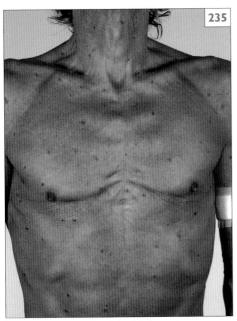

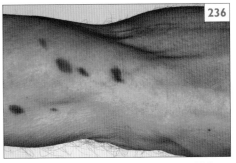

236 Kaposi's sarcoma. Same patient as in **235**. The lesions have a smooth surface and are dark red; some are raised, others are flat.

235 Kaposi's sarcoma. This HIV-positive man presented with numerous red lesions scattered over his torso.

237 Kaposi's sarcoma. Dark, purpuric patches on the legs are typical in endemic KS.

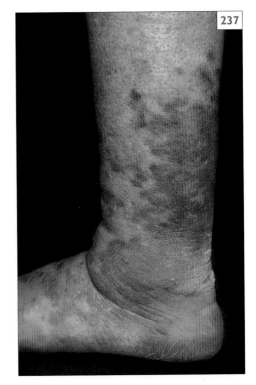

Mycosis fungoides and Sézary syndrome

Mycosis fungoides is a cutaneous T cell lymphoma which can develop at any age but has a higher incidence in the fifth and sixth decades. It generally runs a chronic, indolent course involving the skin alone; however, a few cases progress rapidly with development of cutaneous tumours and systemic involvement. Sézary syndrome is a rare subtype of primary cutaneous T cell lymphoma characterized by erythroderma, generalized lymphadenopathy, and atypical T cells (Sézary cells) in the skin, lymph nodes, and peripheral blood. In a minority of cases mycosis fungoides can be associated with human T-lymphotropic virus type 1 (HTLV-1), particularly in patients from the Caribbean and Japan.

CLINICAL FEATURES

There are four stages of mycosis fungoides. Stage 1 consists of patches or plaques (1A <10%, 1B >10% of body surface area). These lesions have a predilection for the breasts and buttocks, and may have angulated margins. Lesional skin may also demonstrate erythema (with varying shades of redness), fine scaling, atrophy, and poikiloderma (**238, 239**). In pigmented skin the patches can be hypopigmented. Stage 1 lesions can be itchy or sore, however many cases are asymptomatic. Stage 2 has the same cutaneous features as stage 1 but with nonmalignant lymphadenopathy (2A) or cutaneous nodules (2B). The skin nodules (tumours) are firm, indurated, and may become ulcerated (**240**). Stage 3 is erythrodermic skin involvement. Stage 4 is accompanied by malignant infiltration of lymph nodes (4A) and viscera (4B). Sézary syndrome presents with erythroderma and desquamation (exfoliative erythrodema) accompanied by intense pruritus (**241**). Lymphadenopathy is generalized and marked. Clinically there is also peripheral oedema, alopecia, nail dystrophy, and palmoplantar hyperkeratosis.

DIFFERENTIAL DIAGNOSIS
Patch and plaque mycosis fungoides
- Plaque psoriasis (p. 28, scaly plaques in symmetrical distribution, typical nail changes).
- Discoid eczema (p. 14, discrete patches of eczema, usually on lower legs).
- Tinea corporis (p. 154, annular lesions with inflammatory margins).

Tumour-stage mycosis fungoides
- Cutaneous deposit of systemic lymphoma (firm red nodule or plaque).
- Cutaneous metastasis (p. 198, painless red–blue or red–brown nodule).
- B cell lymphoma (p. 196, red or red–brown nodule or plaque).
- Haemangioma (smooth-surfaced red–purple papule or nodule).

Sézary syndrome
- Erythroderma, any cause (p. 51, confluent erythema of >90% body surface area).

COMPLICATIONS
In stage 2 mycosis fungoides, and above:
- Lymphadenopathy.
- Anaemia.
- Hepatosplenomegaly.
- 'B' symptoms: fever, weight loss, night sweats.

In Sézary syndrome:
- Fever, malaise, fatigue.
- Hypo- and hyperthermia.
- Weight loss and malabsorption.
- Lymphadenopathy.
- Secondary bacterial infection leading to systemic sepsis.
- Tachycardia, hypotension, and cardiac failure.
- Acute renal failure.
- Liver dysfunction.
- Thromboembolic disease.
- Capillary leak syndrome.

238 Mycosis fungoides. There are numerous pink, slightly scaly patches scattered on the torso.

239 Mycosis fungoides. Close examination of a patch of mycosis fungoides reveals fine wrinkling.

240 Mycosis fungoides. In advanced disease there are thick plaques and tumid lesions.

241 Sézary syndrome. Sézary syndrome is characterized by an intensely itchy erythroderma.

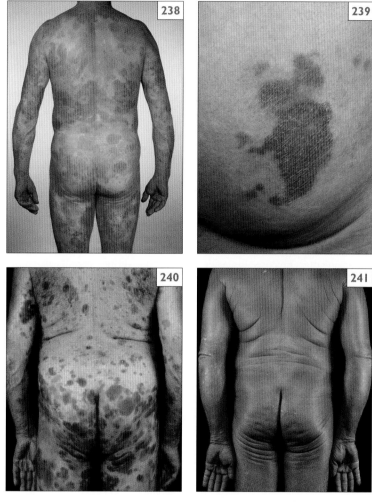

INVESTIGATIONS

- Blood count (usually no evidence of bone marrow involvement until stage 3 mycosis fungoides and above; lymphocytosis is usual in Sézary syndrome).
- Blood film (Sézary cells >10% of total lymphocyte count in Sézary syndrome).
- T cell subsets (increased CD4+ T cells with increased CD4/CD8 ratio (>10) in Sézary syndrome).
- Basic chemistry, liver function tests, calcium, and phosphate.
- ESR (raised in advanced disease).
- LDH (as a marker of lymphoma burden).

- HTLV1 serology (indicating adult T cell lymphoma/leukaemia).
- Skin biopsy for histopathology (mycosis fungoides: infiltrate of cytologically atypical lymphocytes (CD3+, CD4+, CD8-) in the upper dermis displaying epidermotropism; collections of atypical lymphocytes in the epidermis form Pautrier microabscesses; Sézary syndrome: similar to mycosis fungoides but epidermotropism sometimes absent).
- Lymph node biopsy (Sézary syndrome: dense infiltrate of Sézary cells (CD3+, CD4+, CD8-); loss of architecture).

- T cell receptor gene rearrangement studies on skin, blood, and lymph node (if available).
- Chest radiography.
- For suspected Sézary syndrome and mycosis fungoides stage 2A and above: CT scan of chest, abdomen, and pelvis, bone marrow biopsy, lymph node biopsy.

IMMEDIATE MANAGEMENT

For stage 1 disease (which is the majority of patients):

- General emollient therapy.
- Phototherapy (UVB or PUVA).

LONG-TERM MANAGEMENT ISSUES

Mycosis fungoides usually follows a chronic course with a good prognosis. Relapse is common after mycosis fungoides has been cleared and therefore long-term control can be achieved using intermittent courses of phototherapy or topical chemotherapy (mechlorethamine, carmustine). Regular follow-up is essential to monitor extent of the disease. Treatment options for disease advanced beyond stage 1 include: radiotherapy, immunotherapy (interferon), retinoids (bexarotene), and chemotherapy. Denileukin diftitox, an immunotoxin active against cells expressing the IL-2 receptor, has been used successfully in advanced cases. Extracorporeal photophoresis is indicated for Sézary syndrome and erythrodermic mycosis fungoides. The management of mycosis fungoides requires the expertise of a multidisciplinary team led by dermatologists, and including pathologists, specialist nurses, and, when beyond stage 1, oncologists and radiotherapists.

Primary cutaneous B cell lymphoma

Primary cutaneous B cell lymphoma accounts for around 20% of all skin lymphomas. It generally develops in the sixth decade but can occur in children and young adults. Primary B cell lymphoma of the skin is rarely associated with *Borrelia* infection.

CLINICAL FEATURES

Primary cutaneous B cell lymphoma is classified into subtypes: (1) follicle centre lymphoma presents as a solitary nodule or as a cluster of lesions with predilection for scalp, forehead, and back (**242**); (2) marginal zone lymphoma presents as red or red–brown plaques or nodules usually on the extremities or trunk; (3) diffuse large B cell lymphoma – leg type, which is found on the lower leg of elderly women and often ulcerates (**243**); (4) diffuse large B cell lymphoma – other type, which includes a number of cutaneous lymphomas presenting in various ways.

DIFFERENTIAL DIAGNOSIS

- Cutaneous deposit of systemic lymphoma (firm red nodule or plaque).
- Cutaneous metastasis (p. 198, painless red–blue or red–brown nodule).
- Haemangioma (smooth-surfaced red–purple papule or nodule).
- Mycosis fungoides – tumour stage (p. 194, indurated red plaques and nodules).
- Amelanotic melanoma (p. 186, red, fleshy nodule, often with a moist eroded surface).

COMPLICATIONS

Secondary spread is rare but may occur in diffuse B cell lymphoma to:

- Lung.
- Central nervous system.

INVESTIGATIONS

- T cell receptor gene rearrangement studies on skin, blood and lymph node, if available (clonal proliferation).
- Blood count, blood film.
- Basic chemistry, liver function tests, calcium, and phosphate.
- ESR.
- LDH (as a marker of lymphoma burden).

- Immunoglobulins and protein electrophoresis.
- Chest radiography.
- CT scan of chest, abdomen, and pelvis.
- Bone marrow biopsy.
- *Borrelia* serology.
- Skin biopsy for histopathology (follicular cell lymphoma – dermal infiltration of neoplastic follicle centre cells (CD19+, CD20+, CD79a+, bcl-6+, CD5-, CD43-); marginal zone lymphoma – varied dermal infiltration including marginal zone B-cells (CD20+, CD79a+, bcl-2+, CD5-, CD10-, bcl-6-); diffuse large B cell lymphoma, leg type – centroblasts and immunoblasts extending into the subcutis (CD19+, CD20+, CD79a+, bcl-2+, CD10-)).

IMMEDIATE TREATMENT
- Referral to a haematologist for a full assessment.
- Solitary nodules or localized primary cutaneous B cell lymphoma can be treated with radiotherapy or surgery.

LONG-TERM MANAGEMENT ISSUES
Prognosis is generally favourable (5 year survival >95%) apart from diffuse large B cell lymphoma – leg type (5 year survival ~50%). The management of patients with primary cutaneous B cell lymphoma requires the expertise of a multidisciplinary team. Aggressive treatment with chemotherapy or rituximab is required in patients with multifocal or disseminated disease.

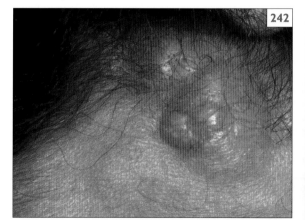

242 Primary cutaneous B cell lymphoma. There is a large infiltrated pink nodule on the anterior hair line.

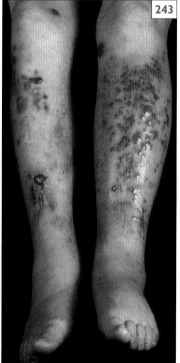

243 Primary cutaneous B cell lymphoma. There are numerous purple nodules on the lower legs of this elderly woman.

Cutaneous metastases

Secondary spread to the skin is unusual in visceral malignancy but when it occurs heralds a poor prognosis. In most cases skin metastases develop months or years after the primary malignancy has been diagnosed; however, rarely, cutaneous metastasis can be the first presentation of an internal cancer. Approximately 60% of skin metastases are adenocarcinomas, usually arising from the colon, lung, or breast, and 15% are squamous in origin arising from the mouth, oesophagus, or lung. Renal cell carcinoma can disseminate to the skin, especially the scalp. Haematological malignancies can also spread to the skin; the dissemination of multiple leukaemic skin deposits is known as leukaemia cutis.

CLINICAL FEATURES

Cutaneous metastases usually occur as a cluster of nodules (**244**) or as a solitary lesion measuring 1–3 cm in diameter (**245**). They are painless, nontender, and red–brown or red–blue in colour. Melanoma metastases are blue–black. The scalp is a common site for metastasis, elsewhere skin secondaries tend to occur on a surface near the underlying tumour, e.g. the chest skin in bronchogenic cancers, the head and neck in oral cavity tumours. Breast cancer may spread to the overlying skin producing a variety of appearances: carcinoma erysipeloides – a zone of warm, indurated erythema (**246**); carcinoma telangiecticum – a sclerotic, telangiectactic plaque; carcinoma *en cuirasse* – noninflammatory skin induration. A metastasis in the umbilicus is known as a Sister Mary Joseph nodule and marks an underlying adenocarcinoma of the stomach, colon, ovary, endometrium, or pancreas. The identification of cutaneous metastasis, in the absence of an undiagnosed primary, necessitates a full clinical examination.

DIFFERENTIAL DIAGNOSIS

- Epidermoid cyst (dome-shaped nodule, often on the scalp, with a punctum).
- Basal cell carcinoma (nodule or plaque with telangiectasiae and a translucent margin; may ulcerate).
- Haemangioma (smooth-surfaced, red–purple papule or nodule).
- Dermatofibroma (firm, red–brown, intradermal papule or nodule).
- Amelanotic melanoma (p. 186, red, fleshy nodule, often with a moist eroded surface).
- B cell lymphoma (p. 196, red or red–brown nodule or plaque).

COMPLICATIONS

Primary tumours which metastasize to skin are:
- Lung.
- Breast.
- Colon.
- Melanoma.
- Renal.
- SCC of oral cavity.
- Myeloid leukaemias.

INVESTIGATIONS

Skin biopsy is performed for histopathology (the lesion is within the dermis; the pathological changes will resemble the primary tumour; lymphatic involvement can be prominent).

IMMEDIATE TREATMENT

Since skin metastases are usually asymptomatic, immediate treatment is not necessary. In the absence of a known primary, investigations must be directed to detection of the visceral tumour. Referral to an oncologist is required.

LONG-TERM MANAGEMENT ISSUES

The presence of cutaneous metastases usually indicates that the underlying cancer has disseminated to other organs. The management of such patients requires the expertise of a multidisciplinary team, including oncology, radiotherapy, and palliative care.

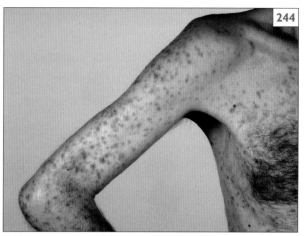

244 Leukaemia cutis. There are numerous red papules and nodules disseminated all over the skin. The patient had underlying chronic lymphocytic leukaemia.

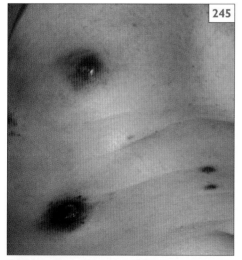

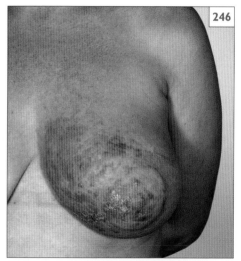

245 Cutaneous metastases. There are two large, red nodules on the torso of this man with multiple myeloma. The skin biopsy demonstrated plasmacytoma.

246 Carcinoma erysipeloides. There is a large area of red, indurated skin caused by lymphatic spread from an underlying breast adenocarcinoma.

CHAPTER 16

Environmental and physical dermatoses

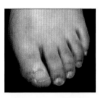 Chilblains

 Dermatitis artefacta

 Miliaria

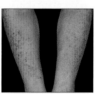 Polymorphic light eruption

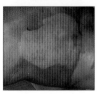 Minor burns

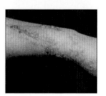 Phytophoto-dermatitis

Chilblains

Chilblains (perniosis) are localized inflammatory lesions which occur as an abnormal reaction to cold. They tend to develop in autumn or winter in countries in which the climate is both cold and humid. Chilblains can be associated with an underlying systemic disorder, including systemic lupus erythematosus, leukaemia, dysproteinaemias, myelodysplasia, and anorexia nervosa.

CLINICAL FEATURES

Chilblains are red–purple papules and plaques which develop on acral skin, i.e. fingers, toes, heels, thighs, nose, and ears (**247, 248**). They occur in susceptible individuals following exposure to cold. The lesions are often itchy but can also be painful and tender. Occasionally chilblains may blister or ulcerate. They tend to resolve spontaneously after a few weeks.

DIFFERENTIAL DIAGNOSIS

- Granuloma annulare (nonscaly, annular plaques and papules, often on acral skin).
- Sarcoidosis (p. 46, nonscaly, violaceous papules and plaques often on the face).
- Erythema multiforme (p. 144, urticated or blistered target-like lesions especially on acral skin).
- Peripheral vascular insufficiency (dusky acral skin, sometimes accompanied by ulceration).
- Small vessel vasculitis (p. 82, palpable purpura, especially on lower legs and feet).

COMPLICATIONS

There are usually none.

INVESTIGATIONS

- The diagnosis is usually made clinically.
- Skin biopsy for histopathology, if diagnosis is unclear (spongiosis, oedema of the papillary dermis, superficial and deep perivascular mononuclear cell infiltrate).
- Blood count, blood film, serum protein electrophoresis and, if appropriate, bone marrow biopsy (to exclude haematological malignancy).
- ANA, anti-dsDNA, -Sm, -RNP, -Ro(SS-A), -La(SS-B) antibodies, complement (to exclude systemic lupus erythematosus).

IMMEDIATE MANAGEMENT

Keep affected body parts warm.

Topical therapy

- Corticosteroid ointment, twice per day (use for a restricted period):
    fingers, toes: potent or superpotent.

LONG-TERM MANAGEMENT ISSUES

If chilblains are developing despite the above measures, consider a calcium channel antagonist, e.g. nifedipine 5–20 mg three times per day, given through the winter months. Warm clothing and heated housing usually stop chilblains. Perniosis in systemic lupus erythematosus may require treatment with oral corticosteroids or other systemic immunosuppressants.

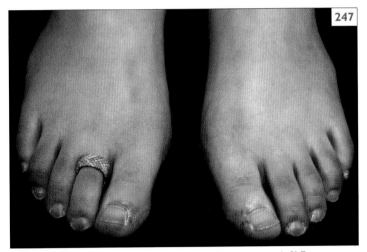

247 Perniosis. Dusky chilblains on the toes of a woman with SLE (chilblain lupus).

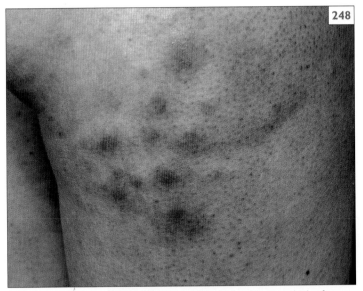

248 Perniosis. Red nodules with surrounding dusky skin on a thigh of a woman who worked out of doors.

Miliaria

Miliaria rubra is a sweat rash which occurs most commonly in hot, humid environments and is colloquially known as 'prickly heat'. It tends to develop after a few months of arrival in a tropical climate but may begin within a few days. There is blockage of the eccrine sweat gland duct which leads to a highly symptomatic eruption when the individual sweats. It may also occur on the backs of bed-bound, hospitalized individuals due to the occlusive effect of plastic mattress covers.

CLINICAL FEATURES

Miliaria rubra consists of myriads of tiny, monomorphic, red papules which occur predominantly on the torso and in the flexures (**249**). In miliaria crystallina there are non-follicular vesicles. The lesions are persistent and produce a pricking discomfort rather than itching.

DIFFERENTIAL DIAGNOSIS

- Folliculitis (p. 120, follicular papules or pustules).
- Cholinergic urticaria (p. 60, transient itchy weals on torso provoked by sweating).
- Grover's disease (p. 50, papulo-squamous eruption on torso occurring in sun-damaged skin).
- Polymorphic light eruption (p. 208, pruritic eruption on uncovered skin induced by sun exposure).

COMPLICATIONS

- Secondary bacterial infection.

INVESTIGATIONS

- The diagnosis is usually made clinically.
- Skin biopsy for histopathology if diagnosis is unclear (keratinization of the intraepidermal sweat gland duct with vesicle formation).

IMMEDIATE MANAGEMENT

Keep affected body parts cool (e.g. cool shower).

Topical therapy

- Emollient therapy.

LONG-TERM MANAGEMENT ISSUES

Miliaria can be complicated by bacterial infection necessitating treatment with antibiotics. Miliaria profunda may follow repeated attacks of miliaria rubra and is characterized by pale, firm, asymptomatic papules. Control of miliaria can only be achieved by keeping cool and reducing sweating. In recalcitrant cases a move to a cooler climate may be necessary.

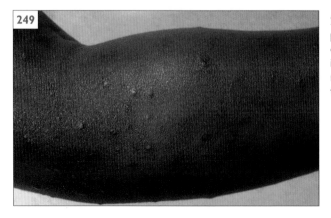

249 Miliaria. Monomorphic papules on the arm which had developed while this patient was in the tropics. The eruption resolved shortly after returning to the UK.

Minor burns

Burns result from a variety of physical agents including heat, chemicals, and ultraviolet radiation. Most burns are due to flame injuries or scalds from hot water. Burn damage causes death of skin cells with loss of fluid through the open wound. Minor burns are painful but associated with only modest long-term morbidity. Extensive (major) burns carry a very significant mortality. The management of major burns is beyond the scope of this book.

CLINICAL FEATURES

The assessment should take into account the source of the burn (flame, scalding fluids, UV radiation (**250**)), other associated injuries (e.g. smoke inhalation), and extent of skin involvement. First-degree burns involve the superficial epidermis only, resulting in erythema and pain. Second-degree burns involve all the epidermis and cause pain, blistering, and a serous exudate (**251**). Third-degree burns cause full-thickness necrosis of the skin and all its appendages; clinically the skin looks pale and there is total loss of sensation. A burn is significant if it is:

(1) full-thickness (i.e. any third-degree burn);
(2) >10% of the body surface area (any depth);
(3) involves the airway, face, hands or perineum.

DIFFERENTIAL DIAGNOSIS
- Fixed drug eruption (p. 228, localized drug-induced erythema and/or blistering).
- Dermatitis artefacta (p. 206, self-induced dermatosis, often in a patient with psychological problems).
- Stevens–Johnson syndrome/toxic epidermal necrolysis (p. 230, mucocutaneous blistering with large areas of epidermal loss).

COMPLICATIONS
With minor burns:
- Secondary infection.

With major burns:
- Fever.
- Systemic sepsis.
- Hypoxia.
- Circulatory collapse.

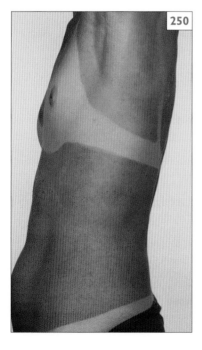

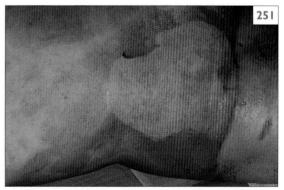

251 Minor burn. There is a second-degree burn on this patient's flank caused by contact with boiling water (scald).

250 Minor burn. This woman received an excessive dose of therapeutic UVB for the treatment of psoriasis. There is confluent erythema over her torso except at the sites protected by her bra and pants.

INVESTIGATIONS

For minor burns:
- Swab for bacteriology if secondary infection is suspected.

IMMEDIATE MANAGEMENT

Assess extent and depth of burn: if it is significant (see above) transfer patient to a specialist burns unit.

Topical therapy

For minor burns:
- Clean affected area with saline or water.
- General emollient therapy.
- Decompress but do not deroof blisters.
- Apply silver sulfadiazine cream to blistered sites.
- Cover denuded areas with nonadherent dressing.

For UV-induced burn:
- Corticosteroid ointment, twice per day (use for a restricted period):
    - face: moderately potent.
    - trunk and limbs: potent.

Systemic therapy

- Give adequate analgesia.
- Administer tetanus vaccine or booster, if necessary.
- Give oral antibiotics if secondary infection is suspected.

LONG-TERM MANAGEMENT ISSUES

First-degree burns heal without any scarring within 5 days. Second-degree burns resolve with scarring and pigmentary change. Appendageal structures such as hair follicles and sweat glands are lost to varying degrees. Third-degree burns for the most part need skin grafting. It is important to document the circumstances surrounding the accident. Burns can be inflicted on vulnerable individuals, such as the elderly, in circumstances of nonaccidental injury.

Dermatitis artefacta

The lesions of dermatitis artefacta (DA) are inflicted by the patient on themselves. The individual is usually fully aware of his or her actions but conceals these from the doctor. The clinical history is often 'hollow' with a lack of detail about the evolution of the dermatosis. DA seems to occur more commonly in young women who, in many cases, are undergoing significant psychosocial stress.

CLINICAL FEATURES

Exposed areas are more commonly involved, such as the face, hands, arms, and legs (**252, 253**). Lesions on the breasts and genital skin are also relatively frequent. Areas difficult to reach, such as the back, are unlikely sites of involvement. DA often presents with signs of superficial damage, such as erythema and blistering, or with evidence of more aggressive destruction causing erosions or ulcers. A variety of physical methods may be used, such as laceration, abrasion, injection, and constriction, which produce a range of injuries. Thermal or chemical injury may also be implicated. The clue to the artefactual nature of DA lesions lies in the bizarre shapes, often with straight lines and angulations, and their monomorphic appearance (**252–254**).

DIFFERENTIAL DIAGNOSIS

- Pyoderma gangrenosum (p. 92, painful, progressive, necrotic ulceration).
- Eccthyma (localized bacterial skin infection causing necrotic eschar overlying an ulcer).
- Panniculitis (p. 102, zone of indurated erythema which may ulcerate).
- Phytophotodermatitis (p. 210, linear eruption on exposed skin caused by interaction of a plant-derived psoralen and sunlight).

COMPLICATIONS

- Secondary bacterial infection.

INVESTIGATIONS

- The diagnosis is usually made clinically.
- Skin swab for bacteriology if secondary infection is suspected.
- Skin biopsy for histopathology if diagnosis is unclear (may show the presence of foreign material within the skin).

IMMEDIATE MANAGEMENT
Topical therapy
- Corticosteroid ointment, twice per day (use for a restricted period) if lesional skin is inflamed and not ulcerated or infected:
  trunk, limbs: potent.
  face: mildly potent.
- Occlusive bandaging will allow most ulcerated or eroded lesions to heal.

Systemic therapy
- Oral antibiotics are indicated if secondary infection is present.

LONG-TERM MANAGEMENT ISSUES
Psychological problems should be approached in a nonconfrontational manner otherwise the patient may disengage with medical services and continue to inflict damage on themselves. Chronic, persistent self-damage requires assessment by a psychiatrist or psychotherapist. Sometimes persuading the patient to see a psychiatrist can prove difficult.

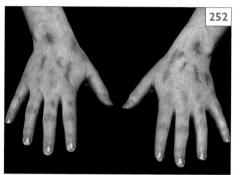

252 Dermatitis artefacta. There are linear lesions on the backs of the hands; some are eroded, in others the skin is intact.

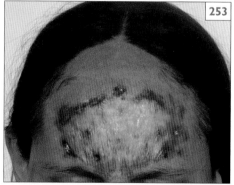

253 Dermatitis artefacta. This woman induced the scarred area on her forehead with a pointed implement, probably a pair of scissors. Note the ulcerated, straight margins.

254 Dermatitis artefacta. A cluster of small haemorrhagic scabs, probably caused by the abrasive action of iron wool or a cheese grater.

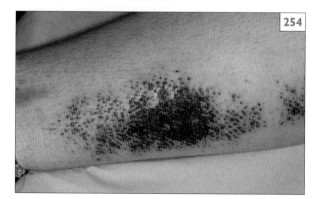

Polymorphic light eruption

Polymorphic light eruption (PLE) is an inflammatory dermatosis caused by a reaction to the UV component of sunlight. Colloquially, PLE is known as 'prickly heat', and can therefore be confused with miliaria (p. 204). The condition generally affects young women and tends to occur predictably when the patient is exposed to strong sunshine. The sudden onset and intense itching of PLE will cause the patient to seek an urgent opinion.

CLINICAL FEATURES

PLE occurs in the spring and summer or develops when the patient is abroad on a sunny holiday. The eruption involves exposed skin only and generally appears within 4–8 hr of sunlight exposure. PLE is characterized by clusters of small, red papules which are intensely itchy (**255**). Other lesions seen in PLE include plaques, vesicles, and blisters (**256**). Not all exposed sites are involved; the eruption most commonly occurs on the backs of the hands, dorsal aspects of the forearms, V of the neck, and legs. Areas of skin habitually exposed, such as the face, are often spared. Following sun avoidance, the lesions of PLE persist for 1–3 days before resolving without scarring.

DIFFERENTIAL DIAGNOSIS

- Solar urticaria (p. 60, sun-induced itchy weals which last for 1–2 hr).
- Subacute cutaneous lupus erythematosus (p. 110, annular and polycyclic lesions on torso).
- Systemic lupus erythematosus (p. 108, rash on cheeks and nose, periungual erythema).
- Phototoxic drug eruption (p. 222, eruption on exposed skin triggered by a photosensitizing drug).

COMPLICATIONS

There are usually none.

INVESTIGATIONS

- The diagnosis is usually made clinically.
- Skin biopsy for histopathology if diagnosis is unclear (upper dermal oedema with a dense perivascular lymphocytic infiltrate).
- ANA, anti-dsDNA, -Sm, -Ro(SS-A), -La(SS-B) antibodies, complement (to exclude subacute cutaneous lupus erythematosus and systemic lupus erythematosus).
- Diagnostic light tests: monochromator and solar stimulator irradiation tests may confirm the diagnosis.

IMMEDIATE MANAGEMENT

Topical therapy

- Sun avoidance and use of photoprotective clothing.
- Use of high protection factor topical sunscreen containing an effective UVA filter.
- Corticosteroid ointment, twice daily (use for a restricted period):
    - trunk, limbs: potent.
    - face: mildly potent.

Systemic therapy

- A short course of oral corticosteroids can clear PLE (e.g. prednisolone 20–30 mg once daily for 5 days).

LONG-TERM MANAGEMENT ISSUES

It is important for the patient to practise careful photoprotection during the spring and summer months and while on holiday. Low-dose narrow-band UVB or PUVA desensitization given in early spring is often effective at preventing or modifying the eruption during the summer. If PLE only occurs on holiday, a short course of prednisolone (20–30 mg once daily for 5 days) can be started as soon as eruption occurs.

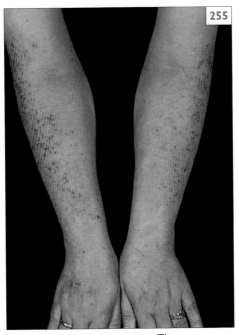

255 Polymorphic light eruption. There are numerous itchy, red papules on the dorsal aspects of the forearms, but not the backs of the hands. Typically, PLE does not affect all exposed skin.

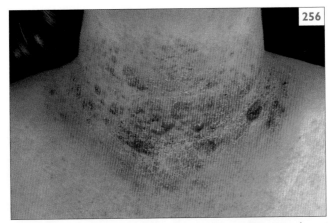

256 Polymorphic light eruption. In this patient, erythema, papules, and blisters developed on the upper chest and neck 4 hr after exposure to strong summer sunlight.

Phytophotodermatitis

Phytophotodermatitis is an eruption caused by the interaction of a plant-derived photoactive chemical (psoralen) and UVA radiation. It usually follows skin contact with culprit vegetation on a sunny, summer's day. The eruption develops with a delay of several hours after exposure to plant psoralen and sunlight. Psoralens are found in many plants including giant hogweed and cow parsley. Other sources of psoralen include celery, lime juice, and oil of bergamot (found in certain perfumes). Tanning lamps emit UVA and can occasionally be implicated in phytophotodermatitis.

CLINICAL FEATURES
Phytophotodermatitis occurs on exposed skin sites which have been in contact with the plant and sunshine, usually arms, legs, and torso. The reaction begins approximately 24 hours after exposure and peaks at 48–72 hours. In the acute phase there are itchy or painful red lesions which may blister. The lesions are often linear reflecting the pattern of psoralen deposition when the plant brushed against the patient's skin (**257, 258**).

DIFFERENTIAL DIAGNOSIS
- Allergic contact dermatitis (p. 18, eczema in a localized area or unusual distribution).
- Polymorphic light eruption (p. 208, pruritic eruption on uncovered skin induced by sun exposure).
- Shingles (herpes zoster) (p. 148, vesicles in a dermatomal distribution).

- Herpes simplex virus infection (p. 142, a cluster of vesicles on a red base).

INVESTIGATIONS
- The diagnosis is usually made clinically.
- Skin swabs for bacteriology to rule out secondary bacterial infection.
- Skin biopsy for histopathology if diagnosis is unclear (perivascular lymphocytic infiltrate with keratinocyte necrosis).

COMPLICATIONS
- Secondary bacterial infection.

IMMEDIATE MANAGEMENT
Topical therapy
- If there is blistering, potassium permanganate soaks.
- Corticosteroid ointment twice per day (use for restricted period):
    trunk, limbs: potent.

Systemic therapy
- A short course of oral corticosteroids can be used in severe cases (e.g. prednisolone 20–30 mg once daily for 5 days).
- Oral antibiotics if secondary infection is suspected.

LONG-TERM MANAGEMENT ISSUES
The acute eruption resolves over several days often leaving marked postinflammatory hyperpigmentation. The hyperpigmentation takes several weeks to fade.

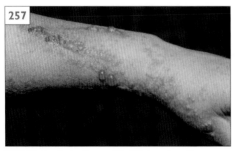

257 Phytophotodermatitis. Blisters in a linear distribution on the forearm of a woman who had brushed against giant hogweed on a sunny day in summer.

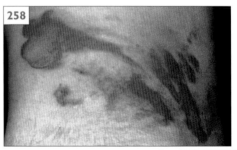

258 Phytophotodermatitis. Large red streaks on the torso, blistered in places, denoting where the patient had come into contact with giant hogweed on a summer's day when not wearing a shirt.

Pregnancy dermatoses

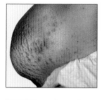

Polymorphic eruption of pregnancy

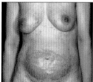

Pemphigoid gestationis

Polymorphic eruption of pregnancy

Polymorphic eruption of pregnancy is a relatively common dermatosis affecting 1 in 160 pregnancies. It is also known as pruritic, urticarial papules and plaques of pregnancy (PUPPP). It characteristically develops in the third trimester of pregnancy (mean time of onset is 36 weeks) and most commonly affects primigravidae. The eruption is very itchy and often develops suddenly, precipitating an acute presentation.

CLINICAL FEATURES
Affected women, who are usually in the last few weeks of their pregnancy, present with an intensely itchy eruption affecting firstly the abdomen and then becoming widespread. The morphology of the lesions is variable; usually red papules, plaques, and urticated lesions (**259, 260**). Rarely annular, polycyclic, vesicular or target-like lesions may develop. The site of predilection is the abdominal striae with umbilical sparing (**261**), however polymorphic eruption of pregnancy may also involve thighs, buttocks, arms, and back.

DIFFERENTIAL DIAGNOSIS
- Atopic eruption of pregnancy (p. 8, flare of atopic dermatitis triggered by pregnancy).
- Pemphigoid gestationis (p. 214, itchy erythema and blisters in second or third trimester of pregnancy).
- Urticaria (p. 55, itchy weals which last for less than 24 hr).
- Scabies (p. 162, generalized itching with burrows in the fingerwebs and at the wrists).

COMPLICATIONS
There are usually none.

INVESTIGATIONS
- The diagnosis is usually made clinically.
- Skin biopsy for histopathology if the diagnosis is in doubt (focal spongiosis of the epidermis overlying a perivascular lymphocytic infiltrate).
- Skin biopsy for direct immunofluorescence to exclude pemphigoid gestationis (negative in polymorphic eruption of pregnancy).

IMMEDIATE MANAGEMENT
Reassure the patient that the eruption will settle following delivery.

Topical therapy
- Corticosteroid ointment, twice per day (use for restricted period):
    trunk and limbs: moderately potent or potent.

Systemic therapy
- Chlorpheniramine 4 mg four times per day.
- In cases with severe pruritus a tapering course of oral prednisolone can be given starting at 20–30 mg daily and reduced to zero over 2 weeks.

LONG-TERM MANAGEMENT ISSUES
The eruption usually resolves at delivery with no sequelae for mother or baby. Most women do not have recurrences of polymorphic eruption of pregnancy with subsequent pregnancies.

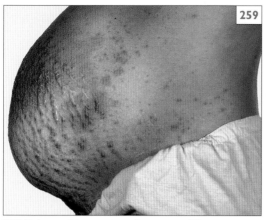

259 Polymorphic eruption of pregnancy. This woman developed confluent, urticated erythema on the abdomen at 38 weeks of gestation.

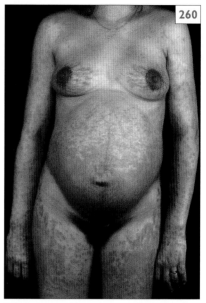

260 Polymorphic eruption of pregnancy. An extensive eruption of itchy, urticated papules on the abdomen, breasts, arms, and legs developed late in the pregnancy of this primigravid woman.

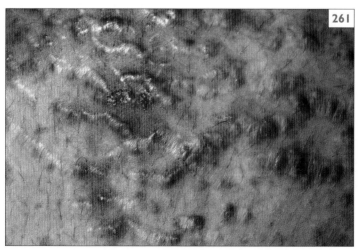

261 Polymorphic eruption of pregnancy. The papules in polymorphic eruption of pregnancy have a predilection for striae.

Pemphigoid gestationis

Pemphigoid gestationis is a rare autoimmune bullous disorder that occurs during pregnancy with an onset usually in the second or third trimester. It resembles bullous pemphigoid clinically and immunopathologically. Blistering is caused by antibodies directed against BP180 antigen and, to a lesser extent, BP230 antigen. Pemphigoid gestationis generally presents acutely as a highly symptomatic dermatosis with striking cutaneous signs.

CLINICAL FEATURES
Pemphigoid gestationis is characterized by pruritic, red papules and plaques which develop into annular or polycyclic lesions. After several days to a few weeks, the lesions blister. Initially bullae develop in the periumbilical area with gradual spread to the rest of the abdomen, thighs, and extremities (**262, 263**). The face and mucosae are usually spared. Occasionally there is spontaneous remission of the disease during the latter part of the pregnancy, only to flare at the time of delivery. Five to 10% of infants born to mothers with pemphigoid gestationis have urticarial or vesicobullous lesions at birth which clear spontaneously within 3 weeks as transferred maternal antibodies are eliminated.

DIFFERENTIAL DIAGNOSIS
- Polymorphic eruption of pregnancy (p. 212, itchy papules and plaques in third trimester of pregnancy).
- Bullous pemphigoid (p. 66, itchy erythema and blisters).
- Linear IgA bullous dermatisis (p. 76, itchy erythema with large tense blisters).
- Epidermolysis bullosa acquisita (p. 74, blisters occurring at sites of mechanical trauma).
- Erythema multiforme (p. 144, urticated or blistered target-like lesions especially on acral skin).

COMPLICATIONS
- Fever and malaise.
- Secondary bacterial infection.

INVESTIGATIONS
- Blood count, basic chemistry, liver function tests (if patient is systemically unwell).
- Skin swab for bacteriology (if secondary infection is suspected).
- Skin biopsy across a blister edge for histopathology (subepidermal splitting with eosinophils in the blister cavity; oedematous upper dermis containing a mixed infiltrate including eosinophils).
- Skin biopsy of perilesional skin for direct immunofluorescence (linear C3 deposition, with or without IgG, along the basement membrane zone).
- Serum for indirect immunofluorescence (circulating pemphigoid gestationis factor in 25% of cases which demonstrates epidermal binding on salt-split skin).

IMMEDIATE MANAGEMENT
Topical therapy
- General emollient therapy.
- Corticosteroid ointment, twice per day (use for restricted period):
    trunk and limbs: potent or superpotent.

Systemic therapy
- Chlorpheniramine 4 mg four times per day.
- With severe involvement a tapering course of oral prednisolone can be given starting at 0.5–1 mg/kg daily. Once the blistering has been controlled then the prednisolone dose can be reduced. If oral prednisolone is required the patient's blood pressure and blood glucose must be monitored closely.

LONG-TERM MANAGEMENT ISSUES
In pemphigoid gestationis there is an increased risk of placental insufficiency, fetal prematurity, and small-for-dates babies. Therefore, the obstetrician needs to be closely involved in the management of a patient with pemphigoid gestationis. If the infant is born with blisters, ensure that neonatal skin care is directed to limiting secondary infection. In the postpartum period a temporary flare of the disorder may occur in the mother necessitating a short-term increase in the prednisolone dose. Warn the mother that there is a high risk of recurrence of pemphigoid gestationis in subsequent pregnancies and that these episodes tend to occur earlier and with a more florid onset.

262 Pemphigoid gestationis. This woman was 25 weeks pregnant. She developed urticated erythema on the abdomen and annular and target-like lesions on the thighs. There is blistering on the right thigh.

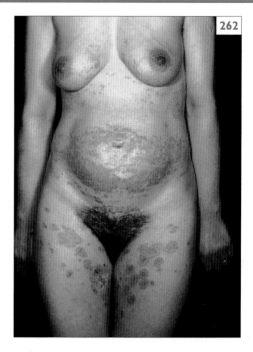

263 Pemphigoid gestationis. Numerous, discrete, urticated and blistering lesions on the arms of the pregnant woman in **262**.

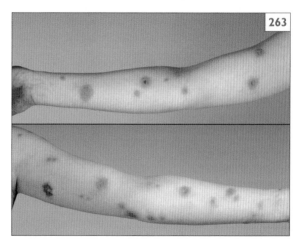

CHAPTER 18

Drug- and therapy-induced dermatoses

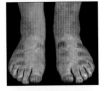 Acute graft-versus-host disease

 Acute generalized exanthem-atous pustulosis

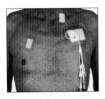 Drug-induced exanthem

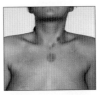 Fixed drug eruption

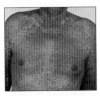 Phototoxic drug eruption

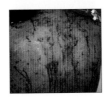 Stevens–Johnson syndrome/ toxic epidermal necrolysis

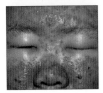 Drug reaction with eosinophilia and systemic symptoms

Acute graft-versus-host disease

Haematopoietic stem cell transplantation (HSCT) is used in the treatment of certain leukaemias, lymphomas, and other diseases of the blood and bone marrow. A graft-versus-host reaction occurs in HSCT when lymphocytes from the donor (graft) are introduced into the patient (host). Donor lymphocytes mount an immunological reaction against epithelial tissue in the recipient to induce a syndrome called graft-versus-host disease (GVHD). The risk of developing GVHD increases with the degree of disparity in histocompatibility between the donor and recipient. Acute GVHD occurs in up to 40% of patients receiving a standard allogeneic HSCT from a fully human leucocyte antigen (HLA)-matched sibling donor; in these cases a graft-versus-host reaction results from differences in minor histocompatibility antigens. Acute GVHD may also occur after transfusion of nonirradiated blood products, infusions of donor lymphocytes, and with solid organ transplants. Acute GVHD is a major cause of morbidity and mortality following allogeneic HSCT.

CLINICAL FEATURES

Acute GVHD is a disorder of skin, gastrointestinal tract, and liver (dermatitis, diarrhoea, disordered liver function tests) which usually develops 1–3 weeks following HSCT, but which can be seen as late as 3 months. The typical rash is a widespread morbilliform exanthem with palmo-plantar involvement (**264, 265**). Thrombocytopenia will often make the eruption purpuric, especially on the legs. Ears, sides of the neck, and upper back are sites of predilection. Other clinical patterns of acute cutaneous GVHD include papular, follicular, and bullous variants. Mucous membrane involvement occurs, especially of the eyes and mouth (**266**). The severity of acute GVHD is highly variable; some patients present with subtle redness of the skin, whilst others develop erythroderma which may be complicated by widespread blistering reminiscent of toxic epidermal necrolysis. Gastrointestinal and liver involvement tends to develop after the onset of cutaneous acute GVHD.

DIFFERENTIAL DIAGNOSIS
- Drug-induced exanthem (p. 220, a morbilliform eruption of pink macules on torso and limbs).
- Viral exanthem (p. 140, widespread morbilliform exanthem with flu-like symptoms).
- Eruption of lymphocyte recovery (rash occurring 2–3 weeks after marrow ablation indicating return of lymphocytes to circulation).

COMPLICATIONS
- Fever and malaise.
- Diarrhoea (gastrointestinal GVHD).
- Liver dysfunction (hepatic GVHD).

INVESTIGATIONS
- Blood count (usually pancytopenia).
- Routine chemistry, liver tests (raised transaminases and bilirubin in hepatic GVHD).
- Skin biopsy for histopathology (focal vacuolar degeneration of the basal layer with lymphoid cells at the dermoepidermal junction; satellite cell necrosis and dyskeratotic keratinocytes).

IMMEDIATE MANAGEMENT

Most patients undergoing allogeneic HSCT receive GVHD prophylaxis in the form of ciclosporin or tacrolimus. Variable T cell depletion of the graft is also commonly used to reduce graft-versus-host reactions.

Topical therapy
- General emollient therapy.
- Corticosteroid ointment, twice per day (use for restricted period):
    face: mildly potent.
    trunk and limbs: moderately potent or potent.

Systemic therapy
- Prednisolone 0.5–1 mg/kg and tapering with response, or pulsed methylprednisolone.
- Increased doses of ciclosporin or tacrolimus.

LONG-TERM MANAGEMENT ISSUES

The damaging effects of GVHD are accompanied by beneficial graft-versus-leukaemia effects, mediated through the same histo-incompatibility mechanisms. Therefore, transplant physicians often attempt to restrict treatment with immunosuppressants so as to strike a balance between GVHD and graft-versus-leukaemia effects. In addition patients with acute GVHD are at high risk of infectious illnesses, another reason to be cautious with immunosuppressive therapy. Chronic GVHD develops in approximately 30% of allogeneic HSCT recipients, usually at least 3 months after transplantation; in the skin chronic GVHD presents as a lichenoid, sclerodermoid, or eczematoid dermatosis.

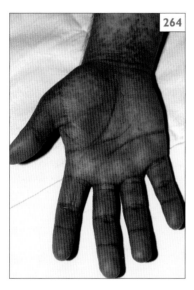

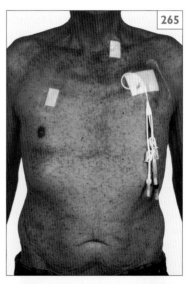

264 Acute graft-versus-host disease. Involvement of the palms and wrists is often seen in acute GVHD.

265 Acute graft-versus-host disease. This patient with acute myeloid leukaemia underwent an allogeneic haematopoietic stem cell transplant. Ten days later he developed a widespread papular and macular eruption.

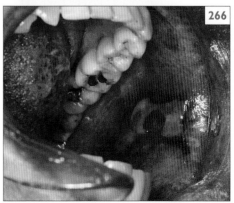

266 Acute graft-versus-host disease. Involvement of the mouth is typical in acute GVHD. In this case there are erosions on the buccal mucosae.

Drug-induced exanthem

Drug-induced exanthems represent a range of cutaneous reaction patterns characterized by a widespread macular or papular eruption. They usually occur within the first 10 days of starting the culprit medication, however occasionally the eruption may not appear until 3 weeks after drug exposure. The commonest drugs implicated are: penicillins, trimethoprim–sulfamethoxazole, anticonvulsants, and NSAIDs.

CLINICAL FEATURES

Typically, there is a symmetrical eruption of small, pink–red macules or papules involving the trunk, limbs, and extremities (**267, 268**). The face is usually spared, as are the pressure areas. Involvement of the skin of the lower legs may be purpuric. Drug-induced exanthems can be itchy but are often asymptomatic. Once the triggering drug has been stopped the exanthem resolves with desquamation in a cephalocaudal manner over 1–2 weeks. However, if the causative agent is continued erythroderma may develop which can become exfoliative.

DIFFERENTIAL DIAGNOSIS

- Viral exanthem (p. 140, widespread morbilliform exanthem with flu-like symptoms).
- Pityriasis rosea (p. 38, an eruption of slightly scaly patches following an initial 'herald' lesion).
- Secondary syphilis (p. 136, papulosquamous eruption with acral involvement).
- Drug reaction with eosinophilia and systemic symptoms (DRESS) (p. 224, drug eruption complicated by fever and significant systemic morbidity).
- Acute graft-versus-host disease (p. 218, morbilliform exanthem with palmo-plantar involvement occurring after a bone marrow transplant).

COMPLICATIONS

- Fever and malaise.
- Lymphadenopathy.

INVESTIGATIONS

- The diagnosis is usually made clinically.
- Blood count (eosinophilia).
- Basic chemistry, liver function tests (if patient is systemically unwell).
- Skin biopsy for histopathology if the diagnosis is in doubt (perivascular lymphocytic infiltrate containing eosinophils).

IMMEDIATE MANAGEMENT

Stop the implicated drug(s).

Topical therapy

- General emollient therapy.
- Corticosteroid ointment, twice per day, (use for a restricted period):
    trunk and limbs: moderately potent.

Systemic therapy

- If itchy, a sedating antihistamine (e.g. hydroxyzine) can be helpful.

LONG-TERM MANAGEMENT ISSUES

Drug-induced exanthems commonly recur on rechallenge, however this depends on the drug and the context. About one-third of amoxicillin reactions develop on re-exposure. The patient should be made aware of his/her sensitivity and should be encouraged to wear an appropriately marked medical alert amulet.

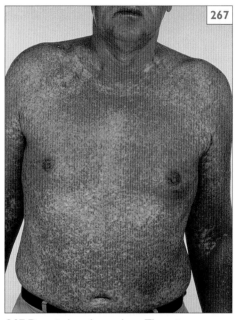

267 Drug-induced exanthem. There is an eruption of monomorphic pink macules scattered evenly over this man's torso. The exanthem had been triggered by penicillin.

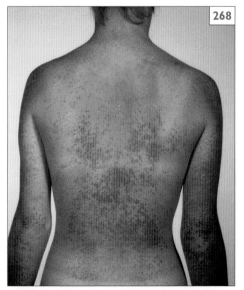

268 Drug-induced exanthem. This patient developed a rash of multiple pink lesions, particularly on her central torso, 7 days after taking trimethoprim–sulfamethoxazole.

Phototoxic drug eruption

Drug-induced photosensitivity can occur in an individual receiving a photoactive drug who is concomitantly exposed to strong sunlight. Culprit drugs include amiodarone, tetracyclines, sulphonamides, phenothiazines, tricyclic antidepressants, thiazide and loop diuretics, sulphonylureas, and NSAIDs.

CLINICAL FEATURES

The dermatosis is confined to the light-exposed areas: face, neck, V of upper anterior chest, dorsal aspect of arms, and hands (**269, 270**). There are several patterns of drug phototoxicity which show variation of time of onset and morphological type. They can occur: (1) immediately following exposure to sunlight causing redness and urticaria; (2) within 24 hr of exposure causing a sunburn-like response (well demarcated erythema with oedema) which sometimes blisters; or (3) within 3–4 days resulting in an inflammatory response and postinflammatory hyperpigmentation. Symptoms are usual and include itching, burning, and stinging.

DIFFERENTIAL DIAGNOSIS

- Polymorphic light eruption (p. 208, itchy papules developing within hours of sun exposure).
- Airborne allergic contact dermatitis (p. 18, eczema occurring on uncovered skin).
- Chronic actinic dermatitis (p. 22, eczema on skin exposed to sunlight).
- Systemic lupus erythematosus (p. 108, erythema on cheeks, nose, and nail folds; systemic features).
- Dermatomyositis (p. 114, violaceous eyelid erythema, Gottron's papules, and myopathy).

COMPLICATIONS

There are usually none.

INVESTIGATIONS

- The diagnosis is usually made clinically.
- ANA, anti-dsDNA, anti-Ro(SS-A) and -La(SS-B) antibodies, complement (to exclude systemic lupus erythematosus or subacute cutaneous lupus erythematosus).
- CPK, anti-RNP and -Jo antibodies (to exclude dermatomyositis).

- Skin biopsy for histopathology (reaction pattern will vary according to type of phototoxicity – usually there is lymphocytic inflammation with variable keratinocyte necrosis).
- Diagnostic light tests: monochromator and solar stimulator irradiation tests may confirm the diagnosis.

IMMEDIATE MANAGEMENT

Stop the implicated drug(s).

Topical therapy
- General emollient therapy.
- Sun avoidance and use of photoprotective clothing.
- Use of high protection factor topical sunscreen containing an effective UVA filter.
- Corticosteroid ointment, twice per day (use for a restricted period):
    trunk and limbs: potent.
    face: mild or moderately potent.

Systemic therapy
- If severe, give oral corticosteroids (e.g. prednisolone 20–30 mg daily and reduce rapidly with response).
- If itchy, a sedating antihistamine (e.g. hydroxyzine) can be helpful.

LONG-TERM MANAGEMENT ISSUES

Phototoxicity can seriously restrict use of certain medications. Once the culprit has been stopped the acute eruption resolves but scaling, lichenification, and hyperpigmentation can persist. The patient should be made aware of his/her sensitivity and should be encouraged to wear an appropriately marked medical alert amulet.

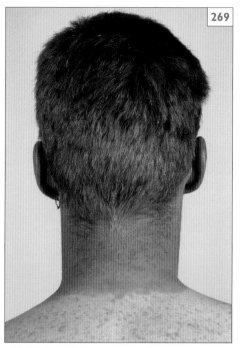

269 Phototoxic drug reaction. A sunburn-like erythema developed on the exposed skin of the neck of this man who was taking ciprofloxacin for a urinary tract infection.

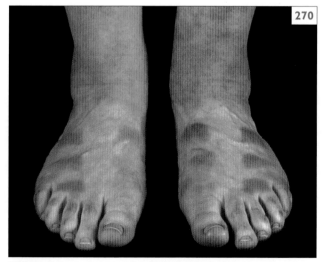

270 Phototoxic drug reaction. This patient had abnormal photosensitivity caused by taking doxycycline for acne.

Drug reaction with eosinophilia and systemic symptoms

Drug reaction with eosinophilia and systemic symptoms (DRESS, also known as drug-induced hypersensitivity syndrome) describes an illness in which fever, rash, lymphadenopathy, and a variety of constitutional symptoms are triggered by a medication. DRESS has a long latency period, occurring 3–6 weeks after initiation of the drug. The commonest culprits are: anticonvulsants (carbamazepine and phenytoin especially), sulphonamides, trimethoprim–sulfamethoxazole, minocycline, and allopurinol. Reactivation of human herpesvirus 6 and other herpes viruses has been implicated in the pathogenesis of DRESS.

CLINICAL FEATURES

The patient presents unwell with a fever and a rash. Sometimes the dermatosis is preceded by a prodrome of malaise and sore throat. The eruption is widespread and itchy, usually manifest as a generalized exanthem of urticated red or purple papules (**271**). Other recognized skin signs include macular erythema, pustules (follicular or nonfollicular), target lesions, blisters, and mild mucosal inflammation. Typically, facial involvement is marked and characterized by oedema (which can involve the whole head), and associated with infiltrated papules and pustules (**272**). The hands may also be swollen. If undiagnosed, patients may become erythrodermic and progress to an exfoliative dermatitis.

DIFFERENTIAL DIAGNOSIS

- Drug-induced exanthem (p. 220, a morbilliform eruption of pink macules on torso and limbs).
- Viral exanthem (p. 140, widespread morbilliform exanthem with flu-like symptoms).
- Angio-oedema (p. 58, large, persistent, deep urticarial swellings, often of the face).
- Acute generalized exanthematous pustulosis (AGEP) (p. 226, drug-induced eruption of sterile pustules with a fever).

COMPLICATIONS

- High fever (>38°C).
- Malaise.

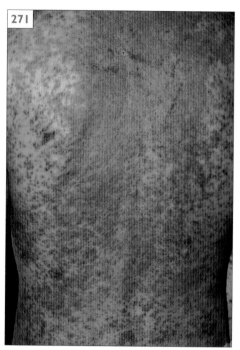

271 Drug reaction with eosinophilia and systemic symptoms. A widespread eruption of itchy erythema and urticated papules secondary to minocycline. This patient also had a fever, lymphadenopathy, and raised liver enzymes.

- Lymphadenopathy.
- Hepatitis (can lead to acute liver failure).
- Pneumonitis.
- Nephritis.

INVESTIGATIONS

- Blood count (eosinophilia), blood film (atypical lymphocytosis).
- Basic chemistry (renal impairment).
- Liver function tests (transaminases usually elevated).
- INR (elevated with significant liver dysfunction).
- ESR, CRP (CRP is usually high).
- Chest radiography (pulmonary infiltrates with pneumonitis).
- Saved serum sample (for drug monitoring/toxicology studies).
- Skin biopsy for histopathology (dermal oedema and a perivascular lymphohistiocytic infiltrate with eosinophils).

IMMEDIATE MANAGEMENT
Stop the implicated drug(s).

Topical therapy
- General emollient therapy.
- Corticosteroid ointment, twice per day (use for a restricted period):
  - trunk and limbs: potent.
  - face: moderately potent.

Systemic therapy
- Give oral corticosteroids (e.g. prednisolone 0.5–1 mg/kg daily) until eruption, fever, and eosinophilia resolve. Reduce the dose of corticosteroid according to response.
- If oral corticosteroids are ineffective or if hepatic involvement is severe, give pulsed intravenous methylprednisolone 500 mg or 1000 mg on 3 consecutive days.

Supportive therapy
Most patients with DRESS will need admitting to hospital for the following:
- Bed rest and intensive topical therapy.
- Initiation of systemic therapy.
- Monitoring of vital signs (pulse rate, blood pressure, temperature).
- Monitoring of liver function tests.

Significant systemic complications (such as hepatic impairment, renal impairment, pneumonitis) should prompt a referral to the relevant specialist.

LONG-TERM MANAGEMENT ISSUES
There is a 10% mortality rate. Unlike a drug-induced exanthem, DRESS can take many weeks to resolve following withdrawal of the offending medication; in this situation prolonged treatment with oral corticosteroids or another immunosuppressive agent, such as ciclosporin, may be necessary. DRESS should be distinguished from the drug-induced pseudolymphoma syndrome, which begins insidiously, runs a chronic course, and is without systemic features. The patient with DRESS should be made aware of his/her sensitivity and should be encouraged to wear an appropriately marked medical alert amulet.

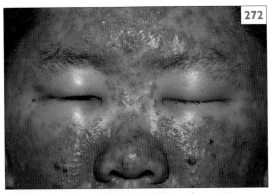

272 Drug reaction with eosinophilia and systemic symptoms. The same patient as in **271**. Facial swelling is common in DRESS.

Acute generalized exanthematous pustulosis

Acute generalized exanthematous pustulosis (AGEP) is a drug hypersensitivity dermatosis characterized by the simultaneous onset of a fever with an eruption of sterile pustules. AGEP usually occurs within 24 hr of exposure to the implicated drug. The commonest culprits are: penicillins, macrolide antibiotics, terbinafine, and NSAIDs.

CLINICAL FEATURES

There is macular erythema, often appearing initially on the face or flexures, covered by myriads of tiny, superficial pustules (**273**). The eruption, which is painful or itchy, spreads rapidly and may become generalized. Involved skin is usually oedematous, particularly when the face is involved. In some cases there are also purpuric or target-like lesions.

DIFFERENTIAL DIAGNOSIS

- Generalized pustular psoriasis (p. 32, widespread eruption of pustules, often appearing in 'waves').
- Candidiasis (p. 158, numerous tiny pustules with desquamation, usually in flexures).
- Sneddon–Wilkinson syndrome (multiple large, flaccid pustules).
- Drug reaction with eosinophilia and systemic symptoms (p. 224, drug eruption complicated by fever and significant systemic morbidity).

COMPLICATIONS

- High fever (>38°C).
- Lymphadenopathy.
- Hepatitis.
- Hypocalcaemia.

INVESTIGATIONS

- Blood count (neutrophilia, often eosinophilia).
- Basic chemistry, calcium, and phosphate (albumin and calcium often low).
- Liver function tests (transaminases sometimes elevated).

- ESR, CRP (inflammatory markers raised).
- Skin swab for microbiology (to exclude candidiasis).
- Skin biopsy for histopathology (subcorneal pustules with a dermal infiltrate of neutrophils and some eosinophils).

IMMEDIATE MANAGEMENT

Stop the implicated drug(s).

Topical therapy

- General emollient therapy.
- Corticosteroid ointment, twice per day (use for a restricted period):
    trunk and limbs: moderately potent.

Systemic therapy

- Give adequate analgesia.
- If severe, give oral corticosteroids (e.g. prednisolone 0.5–1 mg/kg daily) until eruption and fever resolve.
- If itchy, a sedating antihistamine (e.g. hydroxyzine) can be helpful.

Supportive therapy

Admit to hospital for bed rest and monitoring of vital signs.

LONG-TERM MANAGEMENT ISSUES

Once the triggering drug has been discontinued the eruption will resolve with desquamation after approximately 1 week (**274**). Patch testing with the culprit drug may be positive. The patient should be made aware of his/her sensitivity and should be encouraged to wear an appropriately marked medical alert amulet.

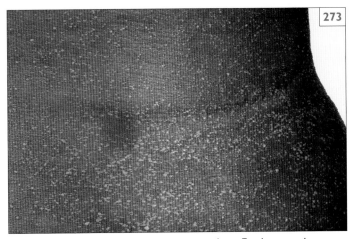

273 Acute generalized exanthematous pustulosis. Erythema and myriads of tiny, superficial pustules. In this case AGEP was triggered by terbinafine.

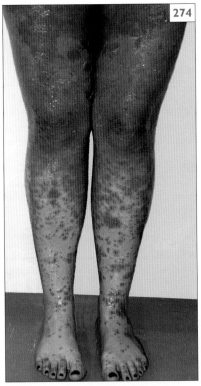

274 Acute generalized exanthematous pustulosis. In this patient AGEP was triggered by erythromycin. The pustules have resolved leaving erythema and desquamation on the thighs.

Fixed drug eruption

Fixed drug eruption is characterized by one or more inflammatory patches that recur at the same cutaneous or mucosal site(s) each time the patient is exposed to the offending drug. Sometimes the eruption has settled by the time the patient consults a doctor, however a history of localized skin inflammation occurring shortly after taking a medication is highly suggestive of fixed drug eruption. Common culprits are: penicillins, tetracyclines, trimethoprim–sulfamethoxazole, aspirin, and NSAIDs.

CLINICAL FEATURES

The typical fixed drug eruption is a deep red, well demarcated, circular patch which develops 30 minutes to 8 hr following ingestion of the triggering drug. Lesions are usually 2–6 cm in diameter but can be up to 20 cm. With repeated drug exposure the lesions may become multiple. Recurrence of fixed drug eruption, following drug re-exposure, usually involves the same site (**275**). If the offending drug is not discontinued the inflammation commonly intensifies, resulting in blistering or desquamation over the following 7 days. Sites of predilection are hands, feet, upper torso, face, and genitalia (particularly glans penis) (**276**). Once the eruption has settled, postinflammatory hyperpigmentation may be prominent.

DIFFERENTIAL DIAGNOSIS

Single lesion:
- Herpes simplex virus infection (p. 142, recurring cluster of vesico-pustules on red base).
- Acute contact dermatitis (p. 18, eczema in localized area or unusual distribution).
- Impetigo (p. 118, red patch(es) with honey-coloured crust, may blister).

Multiple lesions:
- Erythema multiforme (p. 144, red circular or target-like lesions on limbs and acral skin).
- Stevens–Johnson syndrome/toxic epidermal necrolysis (p. 230, mucocutaneous blistering with large areas of epidermal loss).

COMPLICATIONS

There are usually none, unless lesions are multiple and extensive when the patient can develop systemic features similar to Stevens–Johnson syndrome/toxic epidermal necrolysis (see p. 230).

INVESTIGATIONS

- The diagnosis is commonly made on clinical grounds.
- Skin biopsy for histopathology (basal vacuolation, dyskeratosis, and a perivascular lymphohistiocytic infiltrate; occasionally the infiltrate contains eosinophils).

IMMEDIATE MANAGEMENT

Stop the implicated drug(s).

Topical therapy
- General emollient therapy.
- Corticosteroid ointment, twice per day (use for a restricted period):
  trunk and limbs: potent.
  face and genitalia: mild or moderately potent.

LONG-TERM MANAGEMENT ISSUES

Recurrence of fixed drug eruption at exactly the same skin site occurs following exposure to a single dose of the drug, but rechallenge should not be performed to confirm the diagnosis. The patient should be made aware of his/her sensitivity and should be encouraged to wear an appropriately marked medical alert amulet.

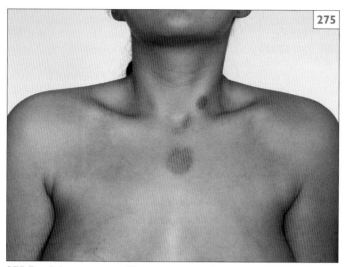

275 Fixed drug eruption. There are two well demarcated, circular macules on this woman's neck and chest triggered by the ingestion of mefenamic acid. The lesions appeared recurrently at the same site on re-exposure to the culprit drug.

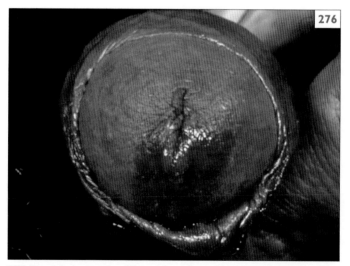

276 Fixed drug eruption. This red patch on the glans appeared shortly after the patient took tetracycline.

Stevens–Johnson syndrome/toxic epidermal necrolysis

Stevens–Johnson syndrome (SJS) and toxic epidermal necrolysis (TEN) are terms used to describe a life-threatening, mucocutaneous drug hypersensitivity syndrome characterized by blistering and epidermal sloughing. In SJS there is epidermal detachment of <10% body surface area, in TEN there is detachment of >30% of the body surface area, while cases with 10–30% involvement are labelled SJS–TEN overlap. Throughout the spectrum of involvement patients suffer distressing symptoms. The systemic problems which accompany widespread epidermal loss can cause serious morbidity, similar to extensive burns. TEN carries a mortality rate of approximately 30%. HIV-infected patients and patients with SLE have an enhanced risk of developing SJS/TEN. Common culprits are: sulphonamides, tri-methoprim–sulfamethoxazole, anticonvulsants (carbamazepine and phenytoin especially), allopurinol, oxicam NSAIDs, and nevirapine.

CLINICAL FEATURES

A prodrome of fever, malaise, and upper respiratory tract symptoms may precede the eruption by a few days. Involvement of the mucous membranes of the eyes, mouth, and nose is a prominent early feature. Eye involvement results in blepharitis, haemorrhagic conjunctivitis, mucus secretion, and pseudomembranes (**277**). Mouth involvement causes an erosive and haemorrhagic mucositis (**278**). On the skin, dusky red macules 1–3 cm in diameter appear at any site and evolve to become confluent (**279**). Atypical target lesions are also seen and, less commonly, typical iris targets (**280**). The skin lesions pass through vesicular and bullous phases (**281, 282**) before epidermal detachment occurs. Shearing pressure to the skin causes detachment

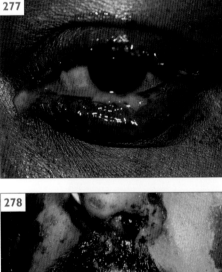

277 Stevens–Johnson syndrome. Conjunctivitis and keratitis caused by nevirapine. The green discolouration is fluoroscein dye used for ophthalmic examination.

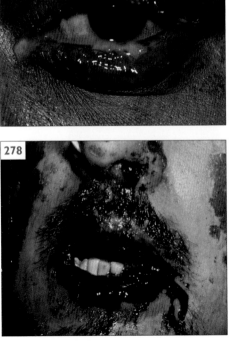

278 Toxic epidermal necrolysis. Severe haemorrhagic mucositis of the nose and mouth triggered by phenytoin. A nasogastric tube has been passed.

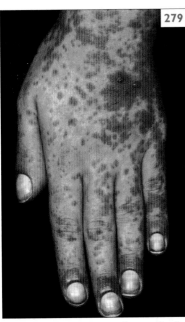

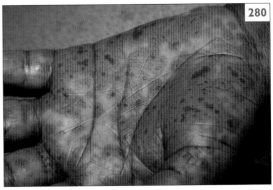

280 Stevens–Johnson syndrome. There are target lesions on the palms. The culprit drug was sulfasalazine.

279 Stevens–Johnson syndrome. Dusky macules on the back of the hand with involvement of the proximal nail folds. There is early blistering. The culprit was carbamazepine.

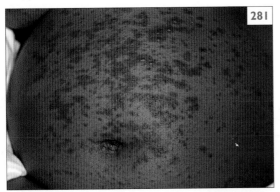

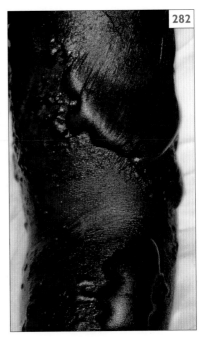

281 Stevens–Johnson/toxic epidermal necrolysis overlap. Numerous dusky lesions which are blistering. These became confluent over the next 24 hr resulting in a large area of epidermal loss.

282 Toxic epidermal necrolysis. Large blisters triggered by sulfadiazine in a patient with HIV infection and cerebral toxoplasmosis.

of involved epidermis (positive Nikolsky's sign) (283). In TEN (>30% of the body surface area) there is widespread epidermal loss and sloughing of the necrotic epidermis which peels back to leave large areas of exposed dermis (284). Denuded dermis exudes serum, becomes secondarily infected and readily bleeds (285). The patient is in severe pain and is usually extremely ill. The loss of an extensive area of epidermis in TEN is associated with 'acute skin failure', a term used to describe the visceral manifestations (see complications) that result from widespread epithelial loss.

DIFFERENTIAL DIAGNOSIS
Stevens–Johnson syndrome

- Erythema multiforme major (p. 144, urticated or blistered target-like lesions especially on acral skin with involvement of mouth and other mucosae).
- Pemphigus vulgaris (p. 68, vesicles, blisters and erosions, usually involves the mouth).
- Mucous membrane pemphigoid (p. 66, erosions and scarring of mucosae with blisters on skin).
- Paraneoplastic pemphigus (polymorphic eruption of lichenoid rash, targets, blisters, and mucosal involvement).

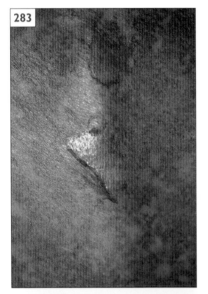

283

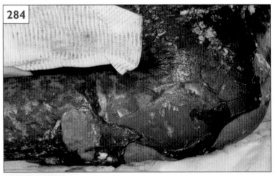

284

283 Toxic epidermal necrolysis. Detachment of involved epidermis by shearing pressure to the skin (positive Nikolsky's sign).

284 Toxic epidermal necrolysis. In this patient large areas of necrotic epidermis became detached. The patient died.

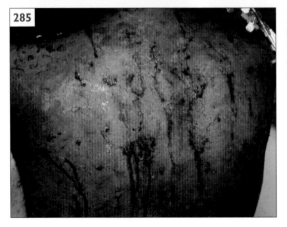

285

285 Toxic epidermal necrolysis. A large area of exposed dermis with multiple bleeding points. The skin re-epithelialized over the next 10 days and the patient survived.

Toxic epidermal necrolysis
- Staphylococcal scalded skin syndrome (p. 134, painful, superficial skin peeling on areas of erythema).
- Pemphigus vulgaris (p. 68, vesicles, bullae and erosions, usually involves the mouth).
- Bullous pemphigoid (p. 66, itchy erythema with large tense blisters).
- Bullous lupus erythematosus (p. 108, blisters in acute lupus erythematosus).
- Linear IgA bullous dermatosis (p. 76, itchy erythema with large tense blisters).
- Generalized fixed drug eruption (p. 228, large, circular, blistered, and desquamating patches).
- Bullous acute graft-versus-host disease (p. 218, morbilliform, blistering exanthem with involvement of palms and soles).

COMPLICATIONS
- Fever, malaise.
- Secondary bacterial infection of skin.
- Thermoregulatory dysfunction.
- Excessive insensible fluid loss.
- Bronchial epithelial necrosis with bronchial obstruction.
- Pneumonia.
- Oesophageal epithelial necrosis.
- Renal impairment.
- Hepatic dysfunction.
- Cardiac failure.
- Insulin resistance with hyperglycaemia.
- Pancreatitis and diabetes.
- Anaemia and leucopenia.
- Thromboembolic disease.
- Septicaemia.
- Multiorgan failure.

INVESTIGATIONS
- Blood count (anaemia, leucocytosis followed by leucopenia).
- Basic chemistry (renal impairment is common).
- Liver function tests (hypoalbuminaemia, raised liver transaminases).
- ESR, CRP (raised inflammatory markers).
- Serum bicarbonate, glucose, amylase.
- Saved serum sample (for drug monitoring/toxicology studies).
- INR, APTT (raised INR in significant liver dysfunction).
- Skin swabs for microbiology.
- Chest radiography.
- Skin biopsy for histopathology (subepidermal blister; lesional skin shows full-thickness epidermal necrosis).
- HIV testing (if appropriate).
- SCORTEN is a specific disease-severity score in TEN composed of seven risk factors for death: age >40 years; heart rate >120 beats/min; epidermal detachment >10%; serum glucose >14 mmol/L; serum bicarbonate <20 mmol/L; serum urea >10 mmol/L; intercurrent malignancy. Each risk factor is assigned 1 point: 1 = mortality rate (MR) of 3%; 2 = MR of 12%; 3 = MR of 35%; 4 = MR of 58%; 5 = MR of 90%.

IMMEDIATE MANAGEMENT
Stop the implicated drug(s).

Topical therapy
- Specialist dermatology nursing care is essential.
- A greasy emollient (e.g. 50% white soft paraffin/50% liquid paraffin) should be applied frequently (every 1–2 hr) to the whole skin.
- Apply topical corticosteroid ointment to purpuric, nonblistered areas (not to bullous or denuded skin):
  trunk and limbs: potent or superpotent.
  face and genitalia: moderately potent.
- Cover eroded areas with nonadhesive dressings and keep lubricated with greasy emollient.
- An antimicrobial topical agent should be applied to eroded or sloughy areas twice per day.
- The mouth should be rinsed with benzydamine mouthwash every 1–2 hr and chlorhexidine mouthwash four times per day.
- The eyes require 1% choramphenicol ointment four times daily, corticosteroid drops (e.g. 0.1% dexamethasone) four times daily and an ocular lubricant (e.g. liquid paraffin) every 2–4 hr.

Systemic therapy

- In SJS, high-dose systemic corticosteroids may be beneficial (e.g. prednisolone 0.5–1 mg/kg daily or IV methylprednisolone 500 mg on 3 consecutive days).
- In view of the enhanced risk of sepsis, systemic corticosteroids are probably contraindicated in TEN.
- In rapidly extending skin loss in SJS/TEN there may be a role for intravenous immunoglobulin, if given early: 1 g/kg daily for 3–4 consecutive days. Evidence for the unequivocal benefit of intravenous immunoglobulin is lacking.
- Ciclosporin 4 mg/kg daily in divided doses may be useful.

Supportive therapy

- Patients require admission to a high-dependency environment, preferably a specialist unit (e.g. burns unit) or ITU, for intensive management and supportive care.
- Assess percentage body surface area of blistered and denuded skin.
- Patients must be nursed in a heated side-room on a bed with an air-fluidized mattress or air-bed mattress. TEN patients need to be handled gently by medical staff to limit further epidermal sloughing.
- Try to avoid using a sphygmomanometer cuff on involved skin – it will cause epidermal sloughing.
- Use 5% lidocaine gel on genital mucosae before inserting a urinary catheter. Fluid replacement should be guided by urine output.
- If at all possible intravenous canulae and central venous lines should be avoided. If venous access is necessary try to use uninvolved skin for canula insertion. Peripheral lines should be changed every 24–48 hr and sent for culture.
- Significant involvement of the mouth will necessitate a nasogastric tube for the delivery of fluids and nutrition. With pancreatic problems or extensive upper gastrointestinal mucosal involvement, parenteral feeding may be necessary. Protein and calorie requirements are high – appropriate nutrition must be guided by a dietitian.
- Monitor skin for signs of infection (pus, slough) taking daily swabs, if needed. Antibiotics must be given if there are direct or indirect signs of infection (tachycardia, fall in blood pressure, peripheral shut-down, falling urinary output, spiking temperature).
- Regular monitoring of blood count, renal and liver function, oxygenation, lung function, and chest radiography is mandatory.
- Anaemia must be corrected with transfusions; leucopenia may respond to recombinant human granulocyte-colony stimulating factor.
- Use low molecular weight heparin as prophylaxis against thromboembolic disease.
- Opiate analgesia is often required for skin pain.

LONG-TERM MANAGEMENT ISSUES

Patients with TEN should be managed by a multidisciplinary team, including dermatologists and/or burns unit doctors, dermatology/burns unit nurses, intensivists, ophthalmologists, dietitians, and pharmacists. Mortality in TEN generally results from overwhelming sepsis or multiorgan failure. Patients who survive the early, critical period will re-epithelialize over 14 days. Ocular involvement in SJS/TEN often results in scarring and can lead to potential sight-threatening sequelae and sicca syndrome. Involved skin tends to heal without scar formation, although loss of nails may occur. Rare, late complications of SJS/TEN include oesophageal stricture, bronchiolitis obliterans, vanishing bile duct syndrome and heterotopic ossification. A drug challenge should not be performed to confirm the diagnosis. The patient should be made aware of his/her sensitivity and should be encouraged to wear an appropriately marked medical alert amulet.

ABPI ankle–brachial pressure index
AC acne conglobata
ACD allergic contact dermatitis
ACE angiotensin-converting enzyme
AD atopic dermatitis
AF acne fulminans
AGEP acute generalized exanthematous pustulosis
ANA antinuclear antibody
ANCA antineutrophil cytoplasmic antibody
APPT activated partial thromboplastin time
ASD adult-onset Still's disease
ASOT antistreptolysin O titre
BP bullous pemphigoid
CA 19-9 carbohydrate antigen 19-9
CA-125 cancer antigen 125
CAD chronic actinic dermatitis
CHOP cyclophosphamide, doxorubicin, vincristine, prednisolone
CPK creatine phosphokinase
CRP C-reactive protein
CSF cerebrospinal fluid
CT computed tomography
DA dermatitis artefacta
DEET N,N-diethyl-meta-toluamide
DH dermatitis herpetiformis
DIC disseminated intravascular coagulopathy
DLE discoid lupus erythematosus
DM dermatomyositis
DRESS drug reaction with eosinophilia and systemic symptoms
DRVVT dilute Russell viper venom time
ds double strand
DVT deep venous thrombosis
EBA epidermolysis bullosa acquisita
EBV Epstein–Barr virus
ECG electrocardiogram
ECM erythema chronicum migrans
ELISA enzyme-linked immunosorbent assay
EM erythema multiforme
EMG electromyography

EN erythema nodosum
ESR erythrocyte sedimentation rate
FDP fibrin degradation product
G-6-PD glucose-6-phosphate dehydrogenase
GPP generalized pustular psoriasis
GVHD graft-versus-host disease
HDU high-dependency unit
HHV human herpesvirus
HIV human immunodeficiency virus
HLA human leucocyte antigen
HS hidradenitis suppurativa
HSCT haematopoietic stem cell transplantation
HSP Henoch–Schönlein purpura
HSV herpes simplex virus
HTLV1 human T-lymphotropic virus type 1
ICD irritant contact dermatitis
ICU intensive care unit
IG immunoglobulin
IM intramuscular
INR international normalized ratio
IV intravenous
KA keratoacanthoma
KOH potassium hydroxide
KS Kaposi's sarcoma
LABD linear IgA bullous dermatosis
LDH lactate dehydrogenase
LE lupus erythematosus
LP lichen planus
MM malignant melanoma
MMP mucous membrane pemphigoid
MMR mumps, measles, rubella
MPO myeloperoxidase
MR mortality rate
MRI magnetic resonance imaging
MRSA methicillin-resistant *Staphylococcus aureus*
NF necrotizing fasciitis
NNN Novy–MacNeal–Nicolle
NSAID nonsteroidal anti-inflammatory drug
PAN polyarteritis nodosa
PCR polymerase chain reaction

PCT porphyria cutanea tarda
PET positron emission tomography
PF pemphigus foliaceous
PG pyoderma gangrenosum
PHN post-herpetic neuralgia
PLE polymorphic light eruption
PPP palmo-plantar pustulosis
PR pityriasis rosea
PR3 serine proteinase 3
PRP pityriasis rubra pilaris
PT prothrombin time
PUPPP pruritic, urticarial papules and plaques of pregnancy
PUVA psoralen-UVA
PV pemphigus vulgaris
RAST radioallergosorbent test
RNP ribonuclear protein
RPR rapid plasma reagin test
SC subcutaneous
SCC squamous cell carcinoma
SCLE subacute cutaneous lupus erythematosus
SCORTEN disease-severity score in toxic epidermal necrolysis
SJS Stevens–Johnson syndrome
SLE systemic lupus erythematosus
SSSS staphylococcal scalded skin syndrome
SVV small vessel vasculitis
TB tuberculosis
TEN toxic epidermal necrolysis
TNF tumour necrosis factor
TPHA *Treponema pallidum* haemagglutinin assay
TPPA *Treponema pallidum* particle agglutination assay
TSS toxic shock syndrome
TSST-1 toxic shock syndrome toxin-1
TT thrombin time
UVA ultraviolet A
UVB ultraviolet B
VDRL venereal disease reference laboratory test
VZIG varicella zoster immune globulin
VZV varicella zoster virus
WCN widespread cutaneous necrosis

RECOMMENDED READING

CHAPTER 1
Allergic contact dermatitis (chapter 13); Atopic dermatitis (chapter 14); Vesicular palmoplantar eczema (chapter 16). In: Wolff K, Goldsmith L, Katz S, Gilchrest B, Paller A, Leffell D (eds) *Fitzpatrick's Dermatology in General Medicine*, 7th edition. McGraw Hill, New York, 2008.

CHAPTER 2
Psoriasis (chapter 35). In: Burns T, Breathnach S, Cox N, Griffiths C (eds) *Rook's Textbook of Dermatology*, 7th edition. Blackwell Publishing, Oxford, 2004.

CHAPTER 3
Parapsoriasis, pityriasis rosea, pirtyriasis rubra pilaris (chapter 11); Lichen planus and related conditions (chapter 12). In: James W, Berger T, Elston D (eds) *Andrews' Diseases of the Skin*, 10th edition. Elsevier, Philadelphia, 2005.

CHAPTER 4
Erythroderma (chapter 11). In: Bolognia J, Jorizzo J, Rapini R (eds) *Dermatology*, 2nd edition. Elsevier, Philadelphia, 2007.

CHAPTER 5
Urticaria and angioedema (chapter 19). In: Bolognia J, Jorizzo J, Rapini R (eds) *Dermatology*, 2nd edition. Elsevier, Philadelphia, 2007.

CHAPTER 6
Immunobullous diseases (chapter 41). In: Burns T, Breathnach S, Cox N, Griffiths C (eds) *Rook's Textbook of Dermatology*, 7th edition. Blackwell Publishing, Oxford, 2004.

CHAPTER 7
Purpura and microvascular occlusion (chapter 48); Vasculitis and neutrophilic vascular reactions (chapter 49). In: Burns T, Breathnach S, Cox N, Griffiths C (eds) *Rook's Textbook of Dermatology*, 7th edition. Blackwell Publishing, Oxford, 2004.

CHAPTER 8
Diseases of the subcutaneous fat (chapter 23). In: James W, Berger T, Elston D (eds) *Andrews' Diseases of the Skin*, 10th edition. Elsevier, Philadelphia, 2005.

CHAPTER 9
Connective tissue diseases (chapter 8). In: James W, Berger T, Elston D (eds) *Andrews' Diseases of the Skin*, 10th edition. Elsevier, Philadelphia, 2005.

CHAPTER 10
Bacterial infections (chapter 27). In: Burns T, Breathnach S, Cox N, Griffiths C (eds) *Rook's Textbook of Dermatology*, 7th edition. Blackwell Publishing, Oxford, 2004.

CHAPTER 11
Exanthematous viral diseases (chapter 192); Herpes simplex (chapter 193); Varicella and herpes zoster (chapter 194). In: Wolff K, Goldsmith L, Katz S, Gilchrest B, Paller A, Leffell D (eds) *Fitzpatrick's Dermatology in General Medicine*, 7th edition. McGraw Hill, New York, 2008.

CHAPTER 12
Mycology (chapter 31). In: Burns T, Breathnach S, Cox N, Griffiths C (eds) *Rook's Textbook of Dermatology*, 7th edition. Blackwell Publishing, Oxford, 2004.

CHAPTER 13
Scabies, other mites and pediculosis (chapter 208); Arthropod bites and stings (chapter 210). In: Wolff K, Goldsmith L, Katz S, Gilchrest B, Paller A, Leffell D (eds) *Fitzpatrick's Dermatology in General Medicine*, 7th edition. McGraw Hill, New York, 2008.

CHAPTER 14
The rickettsioses (chapter 199); Leishmaniasis and other protozoan infections (chapter 206); Bites and stings of terrestrial and aquatic life (chapter 209). In: Wolff K, Goldsmith L, Katz S, Gilchrest B, Paller A, Leffell D (eds) *Fitzpatrick's Dermatology in General Medicine*, 7th edition. McGraw Hill, New York, 2008.

CHAPTER 15
Squamous cell carcinoma (chapter 114); Cutaneous melanoma (chapter 124); Kaposi's sarcoma (chapter 128). In: Wolff K, Goldsmith L, Katz S, Gilchrest B, Paller A, Leffell D (eds) *Fitzpatrick's Dermatology in General Medicine*, 7th edition. McGraw Hill, New York, 2008.

Cutaneous T-cell lymphoma (chapter 120); B-cell lymphomas of the skin (chapter 119); Cutaneous metastases (chapter 122). In: Bolognia J, Jorizzo J, Rapini R (eds) *Dermatology*, 2nd edition. Elsevier, Philadelphia, 2007.

CHAPTER 16
Dermatoses resulting from physical factors (chapter 3). In: James W, Berger T, Elston D (eds) *Andrews' Diseases of the Skin*, 10th edition. Elsevier, Philadelphia, 2005.

CHAPTER 17
Pregnancy dermatoses (chapter 28). In: Bolognia J, Jorizzo J, Rapini R (eds) *Dermatology*, 2nd edition. Elsevier, Philadelphia, 2007.

CHAPTER 18
Erythema multiforme, Stevens–Johnson syndrome and toxic epidermal necrolysis (chapter 21); Drug reactions (chapter 22). In: Bolognia J, Jorizzo J, Rapini R (eds) *Dermatology*, 2nd edition. Elsevier, Philadelphia, 2007.

INDEX

A

acetaminophen (paracetamol) 179
aciclovir 11, 48, 144, 146
acitretin 31, 33, 40, 48, 107, 112
acne conglobata 124–5
acne fulminans 124–5
acral lentiginous melanoma 187
actinic dermatitis, chronic 22–3
acute generalized exanthematous pustulosis (AGEP) 226–7
Aedes spp. 178
alcohol misuse 15, 30, 78
allergens, urticaria 56
allergic contact dermatitis 18–20
allopurinol, hypersensitivity reaction 52
alpha-1-antitrypsin deficiency 102, 103, 104
amphotericin B 176
anaphylactic reactions 56, 57
Ancyclostoma brasiliensis 170
angio-oedema 58–9
angiotensin-converting enzyme (ACE) inhibitors 58
antimony 174
antiphospholipid syndrome 89
atopic dermatitis 8–11
autosensitization 16
azathioprine 47, 68, 71, 75, 116, 144

B

B cell lymphoma, primary cutaneous 196–7
bacterial infections secondary 8, 9, 15, 16
see also named bacterial diseases
Beau's lines 135
benzylpenicillin 84, 128, 132

bilharziasis cutanea tarda 180
biologic agents 30, 31, 33, 40, 71
anti-TNF 47, 92
bites
cat/dog 128
insects 164–5
black fly 174
bladder cancer 115
blepharitis 20
Borrelia burgdorferi 132–3, 196
Bowen's disease 188
breast cancer metastases 198, 199
bulbar muscle weakness 114, 116
bullous dermatoses
impetigo 118, 119
linear IgA 76
bullous pemphigoid (BP) 66–8
burns 205–6
butterfly rash 108, 109

C

calciphylaxis 90–1
calcium channel antagonists 202
candidiasis 158–9
carcinoma erysipeloides 199
carcinoma telangiecticum 198
ceftriaxone 132
cellulitis 126–8
cercarial dermatitis (swimmer's itch) 180
chancre 136
cheilitis, erosive 145
chemotherapy, Kaposi's sarcoma 192
chickenpox (varicella) 146–7
chilblains (perniosis) 202–3
chlorhexidine 118

chlorpheniramine 61, 212, 214
cholesterol emboli 86
cholinergic urticaria 60, 61
Churg–Strauss syndrome 82, 88
ciclosporin 30, 31, 33, 75, 116, 234
cigarette smoking 30, 189
ciprofloxacin 121, 223
clarithromycin 128
clindamycin 123
clotrimazole 159
cold sores (herpes labialis) 10, 11, 142, 143
cold urticaria 60
comedones 124
condylomata lata 137
connective tissue disorders 82
contact dermatitis 18–20
contact urticaria 56
corticosteroids, long-term use 47, 68, 71, 116
crotamiton cream 164
cryoglobulinaemia 82
cutaneous T cell lymphoma 53, 194–6
cyclophosphamide 71, 84, 110, 116

D

danazol 58
dapsone 71, 72, 77, 84, 100
Darier's disease 48–9
dengue 178–9
dependency syndrome 96–7
dermatitis
allergic/irritant contact 18–20
atopic 8–9
cercarial (swimmer's itch) 180
chronic actinic 22–3
erythroderma 51

dermatitis artefacta 102, 206–7
dermatitis herpetiformis 72–3
dermographism 56
desmoglein 1/3 68
N-diethyl-meta-toluamide (DEET) 165
dilute Russell viper venom time (DRVVT) 89
discoid eczema 14–15
discoid lupus erythematosus 106–7
disseminated intravascular coagulopathy (DIC) 88, 90, 130
dithranol 29, 30
doxycycline 138, 223
drug hypersensitivity 226–7
drug reactions
    acute urticaria 56
    angio-oedema 58–9
    with eosinophilia and systemic symptoms (DRESS) 224–5
    erythrodermic rash 52
    exanthem 220–1
    fixed eruptions 228–9
    linear IgA bullous dermatosis 76
    phototoxic 222–3
drug-induced hyperlipoprotienaemia 44

E
eczema
    atopic (atopic dermatitis) 8–11
    discoid (numular) 14–15
    pompholyx 12–13
    venous 16–17, 96, 97
eczema herpeticum 10–11
embolism, cutaneous 86–7
endocarditis, infective 86, 87
epidermolysis bullosa acquisita 74–5
epinephrine 57, 58, 61
Epstein–Barr virus 140, 141
erysipelas 126–8
erythema chronicum migrans 132, 133
erythema multiforme 144–5
erythema nodosum 100–1, 102, 104
erythroderma
    causes 52
    definition 51
    investigations 53
    management 53
    pityriasis rubra pilaris 40, 41
    Sézary syndrome 51, 53, 194, 195

erythromycin 42, 123, 128
    drug reactions 227
etretinate 48
exanthem
    drug-induced 220–1
    viral 140–1
eye disease, SJS/TEN 230, 233, 234
eyelids
    angio-oedema 58, 59
    dermatomyositis 114, 115

F
famciclovir 143, 146
fevers
    dengue 178–9
    rickettsial spotted 177–8
flucloxacillin 9, 12, 16, 23, 48, 121, 128
folliculitis 120–1
foreign body panniculitis 102, 104
Fournier's gangrene 128
furunculosis 120–1
fusidic acid 118, 121

G
G-6-PD deficiency 76, 77
genital disease
    candidiasis 158, 159
    herpes simplex 142, 143, 145
    syphilis 136–8
German measles (rubella) 140
gluten-sensitive enteropathy 72
Gonococcus 130
Gottron's lines/papules 114, 115
graft-versus-host disease 218–19
Grover's disease 50

H
haematopoietic stem cell transplantation 218, 219
haemochromatosis 78, 79
head lice 166–8
'heliotrope' rash 114, 115
Henoch–Schönlein purpura 82
hepatitis B and C infections 78, 82
'herald' patch 38
herpes labialis 10, 11, 142, 143
herpes simplex virus (HSV)
    infections 142–3
    reactivation 144–5
    secondary 10–11, 48
herpes zoster (shingles) 148–50
hidradenitis suppurativa 122–3
HIV infection 20, 30, 78, 82, 192–3, 230, 231

hookworm, dog 170
human botfly infestation (myiasis) 171
human herpes viruses (HHV) 38, 192
human T-lymphotropic virus type 1 (HTLV-1) 194, 195
hydrocortisone sodium succinate 61
hydroxychloroquine 107, 110, 112
hydroxyurea 33
hyperhidrosis 12
hyperkeratosis 28, 29, 40
hyperlipoprotienaemia 44
hyperparathyroidism, secondary 90, 91
hyperpigmentation 38, 39, 100, 101

I
immobility, long-standing 96–7
immunodeficiency 192
impetiginization 8, 9, 29
impetigo 118–19
infectious mononucleosis 140, 141
inflammatory bowel disease 101
insect bites 164–5
intertrigo, candidal 158
intravenous immunoglobulin therapy 71, 234
irritant contact dermatitis 18–20
isotretinoin 124
itraconazole 157, 174, 176
ivermectin 164, 175

J
Janeway lesions 86
jellyfish stings 181, 182–3
jigger flea 172

K
Kaposi's sarcoma 192–3
Kaposi's varicelliform eruption (eczema herpeticum) 10–11
keratoacanthoma (KA) 188, 189
keratoderma 40
Koebner phenomenon 28, 37, 112, 113
Koplik's spots 140

L
Langer's lines 38, 39
larva migrans, cutaneous 170
Leishman–Donovan bodies 174
leishmaniasis 173–4

lentigo maligna melanoma 187
leukaemia cutis 199
leukaemias 92, 93, 94
lice (pediculosis) 166–8
linear IgA bullous dermatosis
　76–7
Linuche anguiculata 181
lipid dysfunction 44
lipodermatosclerosis 102, 104
livedo reticularis 84, 85, 86,
　109
liver disease 78
lupus panniculitis (lupus
　profundus) 102, 104
lupus pernio 46, 47
Lyme disease 132–3
lymphoedema 96–7
lymphoma
　cutaneous T cell 53, 194–6
　primary cutaneous B cell
　　196–7
　subcutaneous panniculitis-like
　　T cell 102, 104

M
malignancies
　associated with
　　dermatomyositis 114, 115
　cutaneous metastases 198–9
　haematological 92, 93, 94
　malignant melanoma 186–8,
　　198
Marjolin's ulcer 188
measles 140–1
meningococcaemia, chronic
　132
meningococcal septicaemia 89,
　90, 130, 131
metastases, cutaneous 198–9
methaemoglobinaemia 77
methotrexate 30, 31, 33, 40, 47,
　110
methylprednisolone 71, 92, 116
microfilariae 174
milaria 204
minocycline 68, 123, 224
montelukast 57
mosquitoes 164, 178
mucous membrane pemphigoid
　(MMP) 66, 67
multiple myeloma 199
mupiricin 118, 121
mycophenolate mofetil 75, 110,
　116
Mycoplasma pneumoniae infection
　145
mycosis fungoides 194–6
myelodysplasia 95
myiasis 171

N
nails
　Darier's disease 48
　dermatomyositis 114, 115
　lichen planus 36
　psoriasis 28
　subungual melanoma 187
　systemic lupus erythematosus
　　(SLE) 109
　tinea infections 155, 156, 157
naproxen 181
necrotizing fasciitis 128–9
Neisseria meningitidis 130
nevirapine 230
nickel 18
Nikolsky's sign 66, 232
nonsteroidal anti-inflammatory
　drugs (NSAIDs) 113, 179,
　181
nose
　lupus pernio 46, 47
　Staphylococcus aureus carriage
　　118

O
occupational dermatoses 18
onchocerciasis 174–5
onychomycosis 155, 156, 157
oral disease
　angio-oedema 58, 59
　candidiasis 158, 159
　Darier's disease 48
　erythema multiforme 144,
　　145
　graft-versus-host disease
　　218–19
　lichen planus 36, 37
　pemphigus 69, 70
　SJS/TEN 230, 234
orf 151
Osler's nodes 86
ovarian carcinoma 114, 116

P
palmo-plantar pustulosis 30–1
pancreatitis 102, 103, 104
panniculitis 102–4
paracetamol (acetaminophen)
　179
paronychia, candidal 158
parvovirus B19 infection 140
patch testing 12, 20
pathergy 92, 93
pedulosis (lice) 166–8
pemphigoid, bullous (BP) 66–8
pemphigoid gestationis 214–15
pemphigus foliaceous 68–71
pemphigus vulgaris 68–71
penicillin 138, 220, 221

permethrin 164, 168
perniosis 202–3
pharyngitis 26, 27, 83
phenoxymethlpenicillin 128
phenytoin 230
phototherapy 21, 29, 36
phototoxic drug eruptions
　222–3
phytophotodermatitis 210
pimecrolimus 20, 21
pityriasis lichenoides acuta 42–3
pityriasis rosea 38–9
pityriasis rubra pilaris 40–1
Pityrosporum folliculitis 120
plant-derived photoactive
　chemicals 210
polyangitis, microscopic 82
polyarteritis nodosa 84–6
polymorphic light eruption
　208–9
pompholyx eczema 12–13
porphyria cutanea tarda 78–9
Portuguese man-of-war 182
post-herpetic neuralgia (PHN)
　149, 150
potassium permanganate 31, 68,
　71, 124
praziquantel 180
prednisolone 57, 68, 212, 214
pregnancy
　generalized pustular psoriasis
　　32
　pemphigoid gestationis
　　214–15
　polymorphic eruption 212–13
　secondary syphilis 138
　varicella zoster infection 147
　'prickly heat' 204, 208
Propionibacterium acnes 124
proton pump inhibitors 68, 71
pruritic, urticarial papules and
　plaques of pregnancy
　(PUPPP) 212–13
pseudofolliculitis barbae 120
Pseudomonas infections 120, 130,
　131
psoralen 210
psoralen-UVA (PUVA) therapy
　29, 36
psoriasis
　erythrodermic 52
　generalized pustular 32–3
　guttate 26–7
　palmo-plantar pustulosis
　　30–1
　plaque 28–30
psychological/psychiatric
　problems 48, 207
pubic lice 166–8

purpura fulminans, infectious
130–2
pustulosis, palmo-plantar 30–1
pyoderma gangrenosum 92–3
pyogenic granuloma 191

R
Raynaud's phenomenon 108
renal failure 90, 91
retinoid therapy 48, 50, 112,
190
rheumatoid arthritis 82, 93
rickettsial spotted fevers 177–8
rifampicin 123
rituximab 71, 74
river blindness (onchocerciasis)
174–5
Rocky Mountain spotted fever
177–8
rubella infection 140

S
sand-flea 172
sarcoidosis 46–7
Sarcoptes scabiei 162
scabies 162–4
schistosomiasis 180
sea-bather's eruption 181
sea-nettles 182
seborrhoeic dermatitis 20–1
septic vasculitis 130–2
Sézary syndrome 51, 53, 194–6
shingles 148–50
Sister Mary Joseph nodule 198
skin fragility 78
skin necrosis
infectious purpura fulminans
130, 131
pityriasis lichenoides acuta 42,
43
widespread 88–90
see also necrotizing fasciitis;
toxic epidermal necrolysis
small vessel vasculitis 82–4
'snail-track' ulcers 136–7
sodium bicarbonate 183
sodium stibogluconate 174
solar urticaria 60, 61
sporotrichosis 176
squamous cell carcinoma (SCC)
188–90
stanozolol 58
staphylococcal scalded skin
syndrome 134–5
Staphylococcus aureus infections 8,
9, 48, 49, 118–19, 120, 121,
134–5
stem cell transplantation
218–19

steroid-sparing agents 68, 75,
110, 116
Stevens–Johnson
syndrome/toxic epidermal
necrolysis 230–4
Still's disease, adult-onset
112–13
stings, jellyfish 181, 182–3
streptococcal infections 26, 27,
130, 134
subacute cutaneous lupus
erythematosus (SCLE)
110–12
sulfamethoxypyridazine 72,
77
sulfapyridine 72, 77
sun damage 22–3, 50, 188,
189
sweating 60, 61, 122–3
Sweet's syndrome 94–5
swimmer's itch 180
syphilis 136–8
systemic lupus erythematosus
(SLE) 82, 102, 108–10,
203

T
T cell lymphoma
cutaneous 53, 194–6
subcutaneous panniculitis-like
102, 104
tacrolimus 20, 21, 47
telogen effluvium 135
terbinafine 157, 227
thalidomide 112
thiobendazole 170
tinea (dermatophyte infections)
154–7
toxic epidermal necrolysis (TEN)
230–4
toxic shock syndrome (TSS) 134
tranexamic acid 58
Treponema pallidum 136
triamcinolone, intralesional 47
Trichophyton interdigitale 154
trimethoprim-sulfamethoxazole
221
tungiasis 172
Tzanck smear 11, 142, 146, 150

U
ulcerative colitis 101
ultraviolet (UV) light 22, 23,
208, 210
burns 205–6
PUVA therapy 29, 36
UVB therapy 21, 29, 36
uroporphyrinogen decarboxylase
78, 79

urticaria
acute 56–7
chronic 57
physical 60–1
urticarial vasculitis 62–3

V
valaciclovir 11, 143, 144, 146
varicella (chickenpox) 146–7
varicella zoster virus (VZV)
148–50
varicose veins 16, 17
vascular cannulation site 93
vasculitides, systemic 82
vasculitis
septic 130–2
small vessel 82–4
urticarial 62–3
venous eczema 16–17, 96, 97
viral infections
erythema multiforme 144–5
exanthem 140–1
herpes simplex 10–11, 48,
142–5
human herpes 38, 192
see also specific viral infections

W
Wegener's granulomatosis 82
whitlow, herpetic 143
Wickham's striae 36
widespread cutaneous necrosis
88–90

X
xanthomata, eruptive 44–5